UN

# Practice Development
# in the Clinical Setting

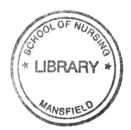

*In the year of their Golden Wedding 2002, thanks to
Stella and Steve for the support they have given to my family.
Rob McSherry*

# Practice Development in the Clinical Setting

## A guide to implementation

Edited by

**Rob McSherry**
School of Health and Social Care, University of Teesside, Middlesborough

**Chris Bassett**
School of Nursing and Midwifery, University of Sheffield

First published in 2002 by:
Nelson Thornes Ltd
Delta Place
27 Bath Road
CHELTENHAM
GL53 7TH
United Kingdom

02  03  04  05  06 / 10  9  8  7  6  5  4  3  2  1

A catalogue record for this book is available from the British Library

ISBN 0-7487-6146-2

Page make-up by Acorn Bookwork

Printed and bound in Great Britain by Ashford Colour Press

# CONTENTS

# Foreword

Practice development must be one of the most enigmatic activities of contemporary health care. At one and the same time, everyone knows what it is and yet nobody knows what it is at all. Within considerably less than a decade, practice development has become fundamental to the infrastructure of NHS Trusts as they strive to meet the volatile policy context in which they operate. Development, or change, is the concern of organisations now and without this they cannot hope to meet the directives of performance management or clinical governance. No self-respecting clinical area or organisation is without a practice development lead!

Job descriptions in practice development vary enormously however. This could be someone who is concerned with the skill expansion of the workforce (such as venepuncture), to someone who is concerned with the implementation of evidence-based practice, to someone who is responsible for whole system development and restructuring of services to meet the needs of service users. It is without doubt this latter job description that I feel most comfortable about when thinking about practice development. My tendency to reject these other job descriptions about practice development concerns the other side of the enigma.

It is actually so very hard to pin down practice development, to define what it is actually about, to describe the impact that it really has on patient care. This book goes a long way to achieving this however. Every now and then, the published word lags behind practice – and developing an understanding of practice development is one of those times. We are only just beginning to see material published about it, yet the role has been implemented with such eagerness in practice. This means that our ability to conceptualise it is naïve and probably incomplete.

We are, however, beginning to appreciate the diversity of activity associated with practice development. Just some of the issues explored in this text are: research implementation; reflective practice; teamworking; leadership; change management; managing barriers; overcoming resistance. I could go on and on! All of this points to two key issues though – thinking and being engaged. This is why I might reject skill expansion or the implementation of evidence, by themselves, as practice development. Both need to be understood in a much broader way as being about helping practitioners and services to better meet the needs of service users. This is not a modest ambition! It is, though, a very exciting process and thinking about and engaging with the content of this book is an excellent way in which you will advance your own understanding of that most essential aspect of professional life, the development of practice.

Charlotte L. Clarke
Professor of Nursing Practice Development Research,
Northumbria University
August 2002

# PREFACE

This text is written in response to key issues highlighted by the Department of Health (DoH) white papers (DoH, 1997; 1998) and *The National Plan* (2001), in which individuals, teams, and organisations are firmly exhorted to modernise. Modernisation means the development of new ways of practising to meet the challenges of the 21st century. In the United Kingdom the paradigm of clinical governance provides an opportunistic framework to help individuals, teams, and organisations working in health and social care to provide efficient and effective services (McSherry and Pearce, 2002). To do this, systems and processes need to be in place which enable individuals, teams, and organisations to develop new and evaluate existing practices so that findings can be disseminated to improve the quality of the service. An essential and often neglected component of the quality agenda in health care governance is 'practice development', that is, the advancement of practice by the development of mutually supportive partnerships between clinical practice, education, and management. This approach enables individuals, teams, and organisations to develop, implement, and evaluate practices on the basis of the best possible evidence.

This book is a comprehensive guide to the introduction of practice development in health and social care. It aims to:

- outline the reasons for practice development;
- describe what we mean by practice development;
- help you develop a strategy for implementing practice development;
- discuss managerial issues pertaining to practice development;
- identify and explore the barriers to practice development;
- consider how to overcome barriers to practice development;
- examine the legal implications of practice development;
- envision the future of practice development.

The book introduces and explores the key issues relating to practice development and aims to enable the health and social care professionals to engage in practice development in their area of practice, working through the obstacles of everyday practice, in their efforts to provide clinical quality. The text employs a problem-solving approach with reflective questions, activities, and case studies.

Rob McSherry and Chris Bassett

Every effort has been made to contact copyright holders of any material reproduced and we apologise if any have been overlooked. Crown copyright material (Activity 6.1) is reproduced with the permission of the Controller of HMSO and the Queen's Printer for Scotland.

# THE CONTRIBUTORS

**Angela Artley**
Assistant Director of Nursing Development at South Cleveland Hospital
NHS Trust, Middlesbrough.

**Chris Bassett**
Lecturer in Nursing at the University of Sheffield.

**Jean Carter**
Clinical Risk Manager at South Cleveland Hospital NHS Trust,
Middlesbrough.

**Deborah Glover**
Editor of the *Journal of Wound Care*.

**Carole Hopps**
Lecturer in Nursing at the University of Sheffield.

**Tina Long**
Lead Nurse at Carlisle and District Primary Care Trust.

**Rob McSherry**
Principal Lecturer in Practice Development at the Postgraduate Institute,
School of Health and Social Care, in the University of Teesside,
Middlesbrough.

**Janice Menhennent**
Practice Development Sister at South Cleveland Hospital NHS Trust,
Middlesbrough.

**Bernie Wallis**
Principal Lecturer in the School of Health and Social Care, at the
University of Teesside, Middlesbrough.

# Introduction to Practice Development  1

*Chris Bassett*

## Introduction

Practice development is an area of nursing and health care that is rapidly becoming an essential part of any health care trust's short-, medium-, and long-term strategy. It is not a new idea; there have been several projects set up to stimulate the development of practice. These projects have taken many different shapes. Some have been simply the introduction of single research nurses or AHPs (allied health professionals) to help people integrate research into practice; some have been the creation of small but dedicated teams with a clear remit to help develop practice in whichever ways were appropriate (Bassett, 1996). The issues are really the same for an individual or a team, being that practice development:

- is an essential requirement for modernising health care;
- is a way to help health and social care organisations, teams, and individuals to improve the quality of the services they offer;
- encourages collaborative partnerships between clinical practice, education, management, and user/voluntary organisations enabling them to develop and evaluate new and existing ways of providing services;
- provides a network for the sharing and dissemination of practices, locally, nationally, and internationally;
- is a valuable way of maintaining recruitment and retaining existing staff;
- though often difficult is achievable.

What we are really talking about when we explore practice development is the integration of research-based evidence into health care.

## Research and health care

The ways in which research findings are implemented into clinical practice are in fact many and varied. However, for health and social care professionals the emphasis is that current and valid research findings should guide decisions about the care they provide to patients. The process of using research findings to guide clinical decision-making is a major factor in providing evidence-based care, as it is known. Evidence-based practice, or the process of providing evidence-based care, is defined as:

> *The conscientious, explicit, and judicious use of current best evidence, based on systematic review of all available evidence –*

*including patient-reported, clinician-observed, and research-derived evidence – in making and carrying out decisions about the care of individual patients. The best available evidence, moderated by patient circumstances and preferences, is applied to improve the quality of clinical judgements (Marsh, 2001).*

It is clear that a care decision that is evidence-based may be derived from several sources of available information. Information sources may include:

- current accepted practice
- patient preferences
- specific patient circumstances
- information reported by colleagues
- practice guidelines
- organisational policy
- government policy (national service frameworks etc.)

When no research findings exist it is necessary to draw upon these other sources of information to reach the best nursing care decision.

## Activity 1.1

How would you decide what to do for a patient of yours who has coronary heart disease? They are sleeping but are due to be turned? Which action would take priority: promoting sleep and pain relief, or promoting oxygen diffusion in the lungs? How would you make this decision? Would you simply follow the doctor's orders? Would you need other information such as the patient's age, respiratory status, vital signs, history of pulmonary conditions, knowledge of whether or not the patient is a smoker, reason for pain, angina, myocardial infarction, degree of pain when awake, duration of pain?

For more information read on and compare your findings with those outlined in the chapter.

Professionals who provide evidence-based care must continually critically appraise all of the available evidence that will help them promote and provide the most positive health outcomes for their patients. Although health care researchers are continuing to generate large amounts of valid and reliable scientific evidence on which to base care decisions, the diffusion of research findings into clinical practice is still lagging far behind the generation of new research findings. Hunt (1981) described five reasons why nurses or indeed other health care professionals do not use research findings. They:

- are unaware of the research findings;
- do not understand them;
- do not believe what the findings indicate;

- do not know how to apply them;
- are not allowed to use them.

In addition to the reasons outlined by Hunt there are several other reasons why nurses and health care professionals are not able to utilise research findings in their practice. Implementing research in clinical settings is a complex process and necessitates understanding of:

- The relationship between the health care system and the generation of health care knowledge for practice, or the structure and process that underlie the research culture;
- the process of planning and implementing change by utilising an established change framework;
- the identification of barriers that prevent nurses from utilising research findings in practice;
- the structures and processes that can potentially enable influence and stimulate an evidence-based work culture.

These four areas (Marsh, 2001) comprise the focus of this chapter.

## EVIDENCE-BASED PRACTICE IN THE UNITED KINGDOM

## Activity 1.2 _____

Where do you think we are in implementing evidence-based practice in Britain?

Do you have any dedicated workers or colleagues who can help you implement research in your workplace, hospital trust, or PGT (Primary Care Trust)?

For more information read on and compare your findings with those outlined in the chapter.

The NHS (National Health Service) has in the past appeared to under-value research, and as a result it is not surprising that the utilisation of health care research that exists has not really taken off. This situation has, however, begun to change in recent years with the publication of several policy documents.

## NHS RESEARCH AND DEVELOPMENT STRATEGY

The NHS Research and Development Strategy was published in 1991 (Department of Health [DoH], 1991) and stressed the overall objective that care in the NHS must be based on research relevant and focused on improving the overall health of the nation. Several subsequent publications of government policy relating to health care and research expressed the expectation that all patient care should be based upon the latest and best evidence available.

In 1993 *Research for Health* was published and this document emphasised the need to ensure that beneficial findings from research are translated into practice (DoH, 1993). The Culyer Report (Culyer, 1994) and implementation plans have resulted in research activity at the trust and regional level. The expectation that all health care should be evidence based is emphasised in three additional publications of government policy: *The New NHS: Modern and Dependable* (DoH, 1997), *A First Class Service: Quality in the New NHS* (DoH, 1998), and *Making a Difference* (DoH, 1999). Together these policy papers set the course for 'services and treatment across the NHS that are based on the best evidence of what does and does not work and what provides the best value for money' (DoH, 1997). One of the most recent additions to research and health care policy, *Making a Difference* (DoH, 1999), was directed in particular towards nurses', midwives', and health visitors' contributions to health care. All of the policy documents clearly state that research must underpin all aspects of nursing and health care; all care must be guided by the best available evidence. Nurses and health and social care professionals must gain the skills needed to interpret and critically appraise research findings (Cutcliffe and Bassett, 1997). This is clearly a major challenge to those of us whose job it is to provide care for patients in the NHS and indeed in the private sector, and is what this book sets out to help achieve. In summary:

- Practice needs to be evidence-based. Research evidence will be rigorously assessed and made accessible. Nurses, midwives, and health visitors need better research appraisal skills to translate research findings into practice.
- A strategy will be developed to influence the research and development agenda, to strengthen the capacity to undertake nursing, midwifery, and health-visiting research, and to use research to support a nursing, midwifery, and health-visiting practice. (DoH, 1999)

The responsibilities of any health and social care professional have changed and increased in conjunction with the expansion of the professional's role. The patient and their families are quite rightly expecting the carer to have the answers and to practise in an efficient, safe, and effective way. With this expectation comes the risk that if the professional does not provide evidence-based care, the patient or their family are increasingly likely to call them to account, either through the hospital or community trust's complaints mechanism, or in the nurses' case via the Nursing and Midwifery Council (NMC) professional conduct committee, or ultimately through the legal system. In line with these changes, education of health and social care professionals has begun to change quite drastically. Health carers' professional education is now fully university based and is becoming very much more rigorous in its approach to the teaching of research. A major part of the health and social care professional's role now includes the use of evidence-based practice to underpin the care and treatment that they provide.

## Activity 1.3 _____

What elements in your professional courses encourage research awareness? Do you need to gain any more skills to help you develop practice?

For more information read on and compare your findings with those outlined in the chapter.

### THE NURSES' CASE FOR RESEARCH-BASED EDUCATION

Over the past 30 years or so in the UK, there has been a growing effort in nursing towards research-based practice. This has helped towards establishing nursing as a true profession. Growing professional concern for the best quality care has matched increasing governmental directives for evidence-based practice to become the norm. Research is seen by all to have become essential in improving and developing nursing care, also aiding in evaluation of care and providing clearer guidelines for practice. This is clearly beneficial to the NHS and to the patient. The creation of up-to-date information and research can be used to change practice, enhance clinical care, and assist in the essential requirement for the reorganisation of care in the rapidly changing world of health care. In addition to the changes in pre-registration nurse education there has been a rapid increase in the provision of continuing education for qualified nurses. This owes in part to the implementation of the Post-Registration Education and Practice scheme (PREP) introduced by the NMC (Bassett and Hopkins, 2001).

### PROFESSIONAL IMPERATIVES

Besides the enhancement of care for the patient, it is considered imperative that health and social care professionals integrate evidence-based care as part and parcel of their ethos and practice, which is cemented by the requirements relating to PREP. In addition to this highly significant innovation many nurses and AHPs are working towards higher academic qualifications such as diplomas and degrees. All of these courses contain research awareness modules as an integral part of the curriculum content. Some use profiles to help the nurse or health and social care professional develop care. This approach can be used to enhance the learning and self-development that can be obtained from this book. A section outlining the development of a personal professional profile is included at the end of this chapter to help you structure your learning needs more effectively.

THE PROFESSIONAL PROFILE AS A DEVELOPMENTAL TOOL

## Activity 1.4 _____

Have you started a profile yet?
    Do you know how to start one?
    For more information read on and compare your findings with those outlined
in the chapter.

### Using a personal professional profile to help you develop your practice

The purpose of keeping a personal profile (all nurses have to keep one, and I am sure other health and social professions will soon have to also if they don't already) is to assist you in maintaining and improving the quality of the care that you can provide for your patients and clients. All nurses, midwives, and health visitors are required by the NMC to keep a journal of development, training, education, and reflection, in order to re-register. The profile is simply a tool that can be used throughout your career in a flexible and creative way. There is no right or wrong way to use your profile, just the way that suits you. There are several reasons to maintain a profile other than to help you develop practice.

### Personal advantages of keeping a profile

A profile is useful because it:

- gives you the chance to assess, evaluate, and reflect on yourself and your career;
- promotes self-confidence and motivation;
- encourages you to apply knowledge to your practice;
- can help in planning a career change;
- helps you with your personal review and personal development planning;
- can be used to prove suitability for a certain role;
- can be used to assemble your curriculum vitae (CV);
- can be used to prove professional development for registration renewal;
- enables you to review your career in a systematic way;
- provides, for those indexing for the Higher Award, material that can be easily transferred to the NMC (Nursing and Midwifery Council) Professional Portfolio;
- helps individuals to claim academic credit in the Credit & Accumulation Transfer Scheme (CATS).

The profile is therefore a way to help you structure your learning and will help you to focus upon how you might be more effective in planning the changes in practice that you want to make. It will assist your ability to reflect, enhance your learning, and provide you with a record containing documentary evidence of the steps you have made towards successful innovation.

## Reflective Practice

## Activity 1.5 ─────────────────────────────

How can reflective practice help with personal and practice development?

Do you practice in a reflective way?

For more information read on and compare your findings with those outlined in the chapter.

## Developing Reflective Practice

At first it may be difficult to see how developing reflective practice can help one to develop health and social care practice. Throughout this book the chapter authors will offer you the opportunity to pause in your reading and think about an aspect of care. They also may ask a question. This chance to pause and think in more detail about an aspect of care is important. This is in fact reflection on practice; however, there is more to it than just pausing to think. Reflecting on practice is an essential part of the health and social care professional's role. The ability to reflect on what we do in our daily work is important. An understanding of our practice can be enhanced through reflection. The idea of reflecting on our practice is for many a new and sometimes frightening one.

It may be helpful to briefly consider the process of reflection. There are basically two levels of reflection. The first is a deliberative reflection. This is the kind of thought process that we go through before, during, and after our everyday practice.

- It allows us to nurse with thought, care, and intelligence.
- It happens at all stages of practice.
- It involves skills such as planning, analysing, predicting, and evaluating our care.
- It allows us to make professional judgements.

The second kind is deep reflection.

- It allows us to ask fundamental questions about the basic way we carry out nursing care.
- It challenges our accepted norms of practice.
- It asks searching questions of the practitioner and their practice.

This deeper type of reflection can help to enhance and challenge our practice.

## REFLECTING ON PRACTICE

By systematically reflecting on our practice a great deal of insight can be gained (Haddock and Bassett, 1997). Use the simple checklist below to break down the following incident and make short notes to refer back to later on.

## CASE STUDY 1.1

During a course run by the university that you attended you discovered some new approaches to how you might care for your patients. You are anxious to share the innovation with your colleagues and get it up and running in practice. After having a meeting with your team, you find they are keen to give it a try. However, the manager of the team does not want it to go ahead. He was on annual leave when you had the meeting and on his return you find he is opposed to the innovation, and it is stopped. What went wrong? Why did he not want it to go ahead? This is a good time to reflect on the problem.

For more information read on and compare your findings with those outlined in the chapter.

## CHECKLIST FOR SUCCESSFUL REFLECTION

Here is a list that you might want to use to help you break the above scenario down to its component parts. Doing this will help you see the stages of the process better. You can of course add more or change it around, as your own needs require.

- Causal/contributing factors. What happened? What was the manager's problem with the innovation?
- What measures could have been taken to prevent the incident and/or subsequent complications – how could you have done better?
- Were the appropriate people involved and at the appropriate time?
- How has the event influenced your subsequent practice? Are you going to try again using a different tack?
- Have you shared your experience with your colleagues?
- What further action is to be taken?
- What are your recommendations?

## A CRITICAL INCIDENT

Another way of reflecting on practice is by making use of a 'critical incident'. But what is this, and how can it help you to develop practice? Benner (1984) describes a critical incident as:

- an incident in which you feel your intervention really made a difference in patient outcome, either directly or indirectly (by helping other staff members);

- an incident that went unusually well;
- an incident in which there was a breakdown (where things may not have gone as planned;
- an incident that is very ordinary and typical;
- an incident that you think was particularly demanding.

When you have chosen your incident, write notes on the following:

- the context of the incident (such as shift time, resources, day);
- why the incident is important to you;
- what your concerns were at the time;
- what you were thinking of as the incident was taking place;
- what you were feeling during and after the incident;
- what, if anything, you found most demanding about the situation.

By breaking down the incident in the way detailed above, you will begin to be able to evaluate the situation systematically and be much more effective in your ability to introduce innovation.

## CONCLUSION

It is clear that all health and social care professionals, whether they work in clinical practice, research, managerial or education settings, must work together to ensure that patient care is evidence based. Providing evidence-based care is one way that we implement research findings in clinical settings. That is where those charged with developing practice must start. Practice developers need to enlist all of the skills and attributes from all areas of practice to succeed in the task ahead. We need to get everyone working together. That is what this text aims to do. This book will systematically explore the steps towards effective practice development. It will consider the following issues in some detail. It draws together the thoughts and experiences of several acknowledged experts in the field, all of whom have considerable experience in developing clinical practice.

◀ **Key points**

- The drivers for practice development are vast, varied, and complex.
- Practice development is about the integration of research into practice: clinical, managerial, educational.
- Practice development should be seen as an integral part of all health and social care professionals' roles, and in the context of lifelong learning and continued professional development.
- Practice development is everyone's business.
- Practice development should be seen as an essential component of the government's modernisation agenda and health care governance.

**RECOMMENDED READING**

Bassett, C. (1996) The sky's the limit. *Nursing Standard* 10(25), 16–19.

Haddock, J. and Bassett, C. (1997) Nurses' perception of reflective practice. *Nursing Standard* 11(32), 39–41.

Hunt, J. (1981) Indications for nursing practice: the use of research findings. *Journal of Advanced Nursing* 6, 189–194.

Marsh, G. (2001). In Bassett, C. (ed.), *Implementing Research in the Clinical Setting*. Whurr, London.

**REFERENCES**

Bassett, C. (1996) The sky's the limit. *Nursing Standard* 10(25), 16–19.

Bassett, C. and Hopkins, S. (2001) *Implementing Research in the Clinical Setting*. Whurr, London.

Benner, P. (1984) *From novice to expert*. Addison Wesley, Menlo Park, California.

Culyer, A. J. (chair) Taskforce on research and development in the NHS (1994) *Supporting Research and Development in the NHS*. HMSO, London.

Cutcliffe, J. and Bassett, C. (1997) Introducing change: the case of research. *Journal of Nursing Management* 5, 241–247.

Department of Health (1991) *Research for Health: A Research and Development Strategy for the NHS*. HMSO, London.

Department of Health (1993) *Research for Health*. HMSO, London.

Department of Health (1997) *The New NHS: Modern and Dependable*. London.

Department of Health (1998) *A First Class Service: Quality in the New NHS*. London.

Department of Health (1999) *Making a Difference*. London.

Haddock, J. and Bassett, C. (1997) Nurses' perception of reflective practice. *Nursing Standard* 11(32), 39–41.

Hunt, J. (1981) Indications for nursing practice: the use of research findings. *Journal of Advanced Nursing* 6, 189–194.

Marsh, G. (2001). In Bassett, C. (ed.), *Implementing Research in the Clinical Setting*. Whurr, London.

# WHAT IS PRACTICE DEVELOPMENT?

2

*Deborah Glover*

## INTRODUCTION

This should be the easiest chapter to write. Essentially, it could all boil down to one line. But, of course, like defining nursing itself, it's not that easy. That is not to say that over recent years academics and practitioners such as Garbett and McCormack (2001), Mallett *et al.* (1997) and Unsworth (2000) have not attempted to define it – it's just that there are as many definitions and interpretations as those who have tried to define it.

Additionally, there has yet to be a definitive job description for a practice development post and there has yet to be a definitive person specification and set of professional criteria that the nurse filling a practice development post must fulfil.

Little wonder then that as the concept and the roles have gathered momentum over the past 10–15 years, their development has been haphazard.

This chapter will explore some of the definitions of practice development, the variety of role content, and some of the models used in organisations to facilitate practice development. It is based on both my personal experience and that of others, and aims to be practical and useful rather than an academic exercise. For ease of reading, I will mainly talk about trusts, directorates, and wards/departments. However, for readers working in the community or the private sector, the concepts will apply no matter how your organisation is divided up.

## BIRTH OF PRACTICE DEVELOPMENT

Chapter 1 has already outlined the social and political reasons for practice development. However, these cannot be seen in isolation. The profession itself has also changed dramatically over recent years and this has spurred the need for practice development.

### Striving for professional recognition

In the late 1970s and early 1980s, nursing began to shake off its traditional handmaiden image and began the long journey towards recognition as a profession in its own right. In the UK, Pearson (1983) and Wright (1989) were the trailblazers for this journey by acknowledging that nurses needed to demonstrate the effectiveness of their practice and its contribution to patient care. Thus they created the first nursing development units (NDUs). These were established as

> *Centres for pioneering leading-edge practice development. In having responsibility for pushing forward the frontiers of nursing knowledge, evaluating and enhancing the quality of care, disseminating knowledge to a wider audience and enabling nurses to develop professionally, NDUs were perceived to benefit both the nursing profession and patient care. (Gerrish and Ferguson, 2000).*

These were seen as so successful that in the 1990s the King's Fund and Department of Health funded a three-year programme, which established over 30 units across the county.

Evaluation studies of these units have noted mixed success. Although they have created new methods of organising care, service development, and research (Redfern and Murrells, 1998), demonstrable patient outcomes have not, to date, been shown in any meaningful way (Redfern *et al.*, 1997).

However, it has been clearly demonstrated that the clinical leader of the unit is crucial. They need to be clinically credible and directly involved in patient care, having authority but free from day-to-day management responsibilities (Christian and Norman, 1998). Keep this in mind; it will be useful in the section on models.

## Project 2000

The face of pre-registration education changed with the advent of Project 2000. The move away from the apprenticeship model to an academic-centred education led to the need for a period of preceptorship in the immediate post-qualification period in order to develop practical and managerial skills in the clinical area.

### Accountability and professional development

No longer do we enjoy the complacency of lifelong registration with no requirement to update ourselves during our working lives; we have to demonstrate that we are clinically and professionally up to date in order to meet the requirements for re-registration. And we have to ensure that, since

> *the practice of nursing ... requires the application of knowledge and simultaneous exercise of judgement and skill ... [it] must ... be sensitive, relevant and responsive to the needs of individual patients ... and have the capacity to adjust, where and when appropriate, to changing circumstances. (NMC, 1992)*

Clearly, these drivers – be they national, organisational, team, or individual – require practitioners to examine their practice and explore ways of changing it in order to ensure the best possible care for patients. As Unsworth (2000) succinctly puts it,

> *The desire on the part of practitioners and managers to develop clinical services and aspects of practice has resulted in the development of an infrastructure to support such endeavours.*

## DEFINING PRACTICE DEVELOPMENT

Unsworth (2000) outlines how the concept of practice development is established in social work, counselling, medicine, and, believe it or not, accountancy (although here it is more of a management process intended to find ways of meeting, anticipating, and identifying client needs profitably).

Unfortunately, in nursing the concept is still poorly articulated. Although I had been in such a post from 1990, by 1994 I still hadn't found a definition of what it was I was trying to do with the nurses I worked with. It didn't help that often the activities the staff were taking didn't produce the immediate or quantifiable results that an audit or a skill-mix review did.

Fortunately, Kitson (1994) was able to describe how practice development is

> *a system whereby identified or appointed change agents work with staff to help them introduce a new activity or practice. The new findings may come from the findings of rigorous research; findings of less rigorous research; experience which has not been tested systematically or trying out an idea in practice. The introduction of the development ought to be systematic and carefully evaluated to ensure that the new practice has achieved the improvements intended.*

This definition appears to focus on research being the driver of change and to suggest that the change in practice will prove or disprove the research theory. This concurs with the notion that in NHS (National Health Service) Research and Development the practice development phase is the implementation of research findings into practice.

The concept of practice development being based on patient need was proposed by Mallett *et al.* in 1997. They highlighted the link between professional development and practice development: both are continuous processes, accomplished formally and informally. Despite this link, the two areas are distinct: professional development is concerned with the skills, knowledge, and values of the individual, whereas practice development reflects how those facets are used to advance quality patient-focused care. Therefore, the individual's professional and personal development can develop practice – and this works the other way too. If there is an organisational or national requirement for some change in practice, the individual practitioner will need to acquire skills and knowledge in order for the change to take place. This is supported by Clarke (1998, cited in Unsworth, 2000), who states that

> *The development of practice is integral to professional care; both care for the individual patient and the systematic enhancement of services and the professional role to meet patient need.*

Garbett and McCormack (2001) acknowledge that practice development at an organisational level is often confused with other activities such as quality assurance and evidence-based practice, and that this makes it difficult for practice development nurses to focus their efforts. This led to the establishment of a concept analysis designed to investigate the use of the term and provide clarity.

Results showed that many respondents felt that practice development was a relatively new phenomenon and that it had more to do with role extension and specialisation or education and training rather than the systematic changing of ordinary practice. They associated it more with individuals and groups (someone else's responsibility) than with a set of activities.

Respondents also felt it was defined in three ways; the development of the practitioner, the development of patient care, and, as in the findings of Mallett *et al.* (1997), a combination of the two.

Thankfully, Unsworth (2000) has identified a 'tentative' list of critical attributes that practice development involves. These make it less nebulous and woolly and provide a framework for the measurement or definition of a development. Practice development involves:

- new ways of working which lead to a direct, measurable improvement in the care or service to the client;
- changes that occur as a response to a specific client need or problem;
- changes that lead to the development of effective services;
- the maintenance or expansion of business/work.

However you choose to interpret it, it is imperative that practice development is viewed on a par with accountability, quality, and caring – integral to practice rather than an add-on that one or two individuals might have an interest in.

## ORGANISATIONAL MODELS FOR PRACTICE DEVELOPMENT

There is no 'one size fits all' model that an organisation can use in order to facilitate practice development (PD). The place of the practice development nurse (PDN) within an organisation will depend on factors such as:

- *Size*. In this case, size does tend to matter. A large NHS trust is likely to be divided into directorates or care groups. This may require more than one PDN to be in post.
- *Strategy*. NHS organisations work towards standards and levels of care outlined by government directives such as National Service Frameworks, the National Institute for Clinical Excellence (NICE) guidelines, Essence of Care standards (Department of Health, 2001). Non-NHS organisations are likely to have developed and implemented their own strategies and standards. However, as in any organisation, these messages need to permeate down to be implemented by all staff.
- *Organisational developments already in place*. These can be at an individual level (appraisal, performance review), unit/directorate level

(business plans, quality standards), organisation-wide level (strategy, response to local population requirements). Where will a dedicated PD person fit in?

- *Resources.* Can the organisation afford one or more PDNs? What is the cost of not having one?

Once these factors have been considered, the model in which PD might take place can be considered. My first taste of undertaking 'practice development' within set parameters was in 1990 as a Sister in the Nursing Practice Group (NPG) at the Westminster Hospital, London. This group had developed as a result of project work undertaken on nursing models and documentation. This led to the realisation that there were other issues in nursing practice that could be explored. Fortunately, the organisation had the foresight to realise that it had started a ball rolling and so put a team in place to run with it.

The NPG was based on a trust-wide remit model (see Figure 2.1). Here, the individual PDN (or group of PDNs) sits within the Director of Nursing's team, or the Quality/Clinical Governance department. They then work across the whole organisation, dividing their work between directorates/departments. There is no line management responsibility for directorate staff.

Our NPG comprised three PDNs, each of whom had a specific directorate/unit to work with, according to interest and expertise. I also had a remit to introduce a pressure ulcer prevention and management policy across the trust, so I worked across the whole organisation as well as with the wards I was allocated to.

### Figure 2.1

Practice development nurse positions within a trust board

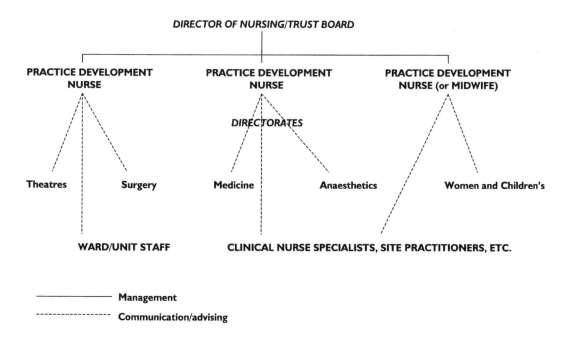

---
Management

---------------- Communication/advising

This model has several advantages:

- The developments take place to meet both the objectives and strategy of the organisation as a whole and those of the directorate. This also allows for local team (ward/unit) ideas to be developed and implemented and their effect in the directorate and organisation to be evaluated.
- Any developments are coordinated. Within a group, PDNs can discuss the issues they are working on at a team level and how they might be implemented across the organisation if appropriate. There is an umbrella view of how, for example, national directives or the organisation's strategy are being received and implemented. The PDNs can also liaise with other staff outside organisation units, such as clinical nurse specialists, lecturer practitioners, and site managers.
- Practice development nurses can build strong relationships with the staff in their directorate. Because they spend a lot of time working with practitioners at ward level, they appreciate the environment they are working in and can help them find ways of developing practice within its constraints. This is much more effective than struggling to react to a voice from above telling them that 'such and such' guidelines have to be in place, by this time and in this way, and then finding themselves in trouble when they haven't been able to comply. The PDN can also liaise with managers about barriers to developments.
- Other team members can cover workload during absences, so that developments aren't suspended.
- Practice development nurses do not usually have line management responsibility for directorate staff. This means that although at times when you go on the ward you may be seen as a pain in the nether regions, you aren't seen as 'one of them'.

Disadvantages include:

- Practice development nurses do not usually have line management responsibility for directorate staff. No, this isn't a misprint. The very nature of change and development means that it can be a long, slow, drawn-out process. Inevitably, when there are clinical or financial pressures, developments get put on hold as being too costly, or 'not a priority'. This is when line management would be useful, since the 'I'm your boss and I'm telling you to do it' approach would be so useful.
- It takes a long time to build trust with staff. Management are often seen as the enemy, rather than part of the team, and the PDN working at trust or management level may be viewed with some suspicion: 'Is she just checking up on my practice? Is she watching how I run the ward? Does this mean staff/resources are going to be taken?'
- Generally, the directorate management team will not have employed the PDN, nor do they manage them. Therefore, they may feel that

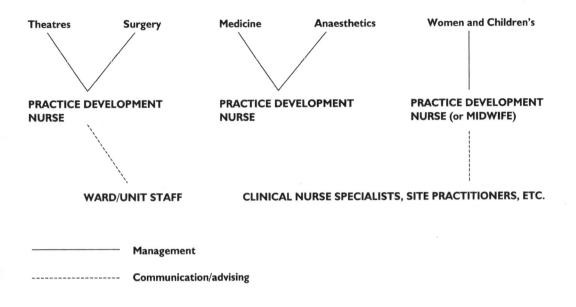

**DIRECTORATES**

Management

Communication/advising

the PDN is there to drive through the organisational agenda, rather than the directorate one.

The nature of the post is, on the whole, advisory. This means that people don't have to accept your advice.

The other model frequently used is where the PDN is based within a directorate or department (see Figure 2.2). Again, this has both advantages and disadvantages.

**Figure 2.2**

Practice development nurse positions within a directorate

## Advantages

- The developments take place to meet the objectives and strategy of the directorate. There is a greater emphasis on local team (ward/unit) ideas being developed, implemented, and evaluated and their effect on the directorate evaluated.
- Developments are coordinated across clinical areas in the directorate and the pace of implementation is more controllable.
- Again, the PDN can build strong relationships with staff in their directorate, especially since they have more time to spend with them.
- Team ideas can be worked on more readily, since the PDN has a smaller workload.
- PDNs do not usually have line management responsibility for directorate staff (see above).

## Disadvantages

- Directorate managers may focus too much on the development needs of their area to the detriment of organisational or national directives.

- There may be a danger of parochialism and a reluctance to share practice.
- No cover for absence. Developments may lose momentum.
- The PDN may become isolated.

Whichever model is chosen, it has to be acknowledged that development is linked at all levels of the organisation – it will not be effective in isolation (Table 2.1). An individual who develops personally and professionally will influence the team. The team's collective developments in practice will ensure quality care for patients. The organisation will concentrate on ways to implement policy and standards and provide the culture and resources to support staff in this.

**Table 2.1**

Practice development links

| Level | Role of PDN | Results |
|-------|-------------|---------|
| Individual | Helping staff with their personal development plans | Active participants and reflective practitioners |
| Directorate | Works in a defined area and with teams | All teams in the units are change agents and receptive to developments |
| | Works within defined resources | |
| | Evaluates developments | Continuing improvements in care, ways of working, and dissemination of developments |
| Organisation | To establish accountability | Local developments can influence organisational developments as appropriate |
| | Works at both organisational and directorate level ensuring developments from grassroots integrate into national or organisational objectives and existing structures | Culture positive to change and adaptation |
| | | Staff feel valued |
| | | Better patient outcomes |
| | | Input into regional and national initiatives |

## PRACTICE DEVELOPMENT ROLES

Practice development roles are as varied in remit and structure as the definitions of practice development itself. One could argue that many posts that do not have the words 'practice development' in their title – Clinical Nurse Specialist, Nurse Practitioner, Clinical Nurse Practitioner, Nurse Consultant, etc. – are, theoretically, practice development roles. However, I believe that they are fundamentally different from the practice development role as I know it in that their remit is usually very specific. Some posts have been established to pick up the fallout from the reduction in junior doctor hours (night/site practitioners) and others, although post-holders tend to vigorously deny it, have followed the medical model and concentrated on one system or part of the human anatomy (clinical nurse specialists, nurse consultants, nurse endoscopists). Although these roles undoubtedly offer easily measurable benefits and outcomes for patients, the post-holder, and the organisation, such as reduced waiting times, personal skills acquisition, and reductions in human resource costs, they do not tend to offer nurses *per se* anything.

Practice development roles, no matter how varied, are all based on the fundamental premise that they exist to help as many nursing staff as possible develop their practice as a team in order to bring about personal, professional, organisational, and patient benefit. The downside being that it all takes so much longer.

## Role content

As I mentioned at the beginning of this chapter, there has yet to be a definitive job description for this type of role. I held three practice development roles between 1990 and 1994 and, although they had some similar elements, in essence they were entirely different. Even a cursory glance through extant job descriptions shows a massive variety of components to the role: auditing, report writing, assisting nurses set up and manage practice development projects, standard setting and monitoring, data collection, coordinating implementation of trust nursing strategy, facilitating staff to meet PREP (Post-Registration Education and Practice scheme) requirements, clinical supervision, advising Director of Nursing on nursing/quality issues that need to be taken to the board, providing leadership to nurses in the directorate, reviewing current practice against acknowledged research-based practice and so on.

The reality is that practice development roles have to be adaptable to the needs of the organisation, directorate, or individual. Most tend to be a 'suck it and see' kind of job, which has its rewards and its disasters.

Mallett *et al.* (1997) surveyed a sample of members of the Professional and Practice Development Nurses' Forum (now the Practice Development Forum – Box 2.1) to ascertain their perceptions of their roles. The results showed how multifaceted they were and included:

- conducting formal teaching sessions;
- dissemination of information from trust level;
- identification and support of individual nurses' educational and development needs;
- resources for professional advice;
- interpreting, summarising, and dissemination of policy documents;
- determining policies and guidelines;
- introduction and support of evidence-based practice;
- liaison with educational providers;
- working on nursing documentation.

There was some mixed response to having to assist in skill-mix and other management issues, acting as a credible clinical role model, and developing patient information leaflets. This brings up two pertinent

**Box 2.1**

In 1994, in my third practice development role, I set up the Professional and Practice Development Nurses' Forum (PPDNF, now the Practice Development Forum). Initially, the idea was to provide peer support for nurses working within this type of role, and to attempt to clarify it. However, at the first meeting we found that we were each facing similar problems:

- The practice development role was often marginalised by operational aspects of the role.
- Both managers and nursing staff required justification of practice development and having a dedicated practice development nurse.
- The levels at which post-holders operated varied. Some worked at grade F; some were on senior management scales. Some worked in directorates; others worked at a strategic level. Some worked alone; others were part of a team.
- Many felt isolated in their role.

Out of these fell the aims of the PPDNF: to chAHPion the role of the PDN, to demonstrate the financial, tangible, and intangible value of practice development for the delivery of nursing care, to highlight the cost of not having such a post, and to provide peer support and the sharing of good practice through benchmarking and an annual conference.

Several years on, the PPDNF has a new name but is still going strong. It has almost 500 members from all over the UK. Four regional groups disseminate the work of the national forum and collect the views of regional members to provide a two-way dialogue.

The Foundation of Nursing Studies is an independent, registered charity with a remit to bridge the gap between research and health care delivery. Today this remit has been strengthened by the increased emphasis placed on evidence-based health care and on the role of practice development as a concept and activity that facilitates practice change and the use of knowledge, research, and evidence

**Support**

For the past seven years, the Foundation has supported the Practice Development Forum (PDF). The Forum aims to 'advance practice development in order to promote high quality client-focused health care'. The Foundation's commitment to facilitating development and encouraging collaboration has enabled the forum to work towards achieving its aim by supporting and promoting roles that develop practice, clinical effectiveness, and evidence-based practice. We believe offering this external support is essential to groups like the PDF and in some way models the kind of effective working that is needed to foster a culture in organisations that promotes effective nursing practice and enables development and innovation. As an independent forum, the PDF also has a key role to play in contributing to and influencing the direction of local and national agendas. Encouraging this independence is another way in which the Foundation can help practice developers to think and be more politically aware and is again a characteristic essential for effective change and development of health care practice.

questions: should PDNs have an operational function and do they have to be clinically credible? I would argue no to both.

## Operational responsibility

Mallett *et al.* (1997) reported that those with operational responsibilities often found that these impinged on time available for practice development activities. Such responsibilities also potentially create mistrust. It is easy to understand why the PDN would be expected to undertake some operational tasks. A skill-mix review, for example, can provide information about the team in order to explore the best way to implement change or introduce new practice. However, having responsibility for the agency nurse budget or bed management, is likely to be time consuming and moves the PDN into enemy territory.

## Clinical credibility

It would seem eminently sensible that a PDN working with practitioners at a clinical level should be 'clinically credible'. I say, leave that to the clinical nurse specialists and nurse consultants. There are two good reasons why a specialist clinical knowledge is unnecessary:

- The post-holder is never going to be that clever! A single PDN working across a trust is unlikely to have experienced all the clinical areas they are covering, let alone have an in-depth knowledge about them all. This equally applies to those working within a single directorate.
- The practitioners working in their ward or department are the credible clinical specialists. The PDN's role is to facilitate the development of their knowledge and skills to improve practice and patient care. Credibility comes from working alongside practitioners in that area, understanding their personal and team needs, assessing the context in which they are working, and helping explore ways that developments can take place or policies can be implemented.

Garbett and McCormack (2001), however, found that the perception of clinical credibility was a factor in staff perceptions of PDNs. Respondents viewed as positive the fact that practice development staff had previously been senior nurses in the clinical area, since they had experience of 'both sides of the fence'. Not having credibility created scepticism about the post-holders, since they 'lacked the necessary expertise and experience to command respect from their colleagues'. It is unclear from the study which type of practice development post was being discussed.

There is also wide variation in the grade of the job. Anecdotal evidence suggests that those PDNs working within directorates tended to be at grade F or G level, whereas those working at organisational level were usually on an H or I grade.

Those working at lower grades often found it difficult to work with ward managers and team leaders, since the latter were on higher grades and perhaps perceived the PDN to be subordinate. A possible solution to this is to take PDNs off the clinical grading scale and use a management scale, although this is likely to create its own problems. Qualifications held by post-holders also vary. Some have post-registration clinical qualifications; others have degrees.

Whatever the components of the post and the skills and knowledge required of the post-holder, practice development should be seen as a long-term investment. Results rarely happen in the first few months. The following issues will influence progress, so they are worth assessing and discussing with both managers and staff at all levels.

### The current practice development / research culture within the organisation.

- Are developments encouraged by managers?
- What perceptions do practitioners hold about research and practice development (especially research)? What do they know about it? Is it scary? Is it something that only the medics are encouraged to do?
- Who generates / has generated any current developments?
- Existing practice: good, poor, indifferent (we've always done it this way), based on best evidence or custom and local policies?

### Staffing establishment and skill mix

- Does each ward/unit have an establishment that will support staff to take time out in order to consider practice developments and obtain the requisite skills?
- Does the ward/unit manager have the skills to influence/support / undertake/facilitate developments and research?
- Can support staff be included in the developments? What are their training needs if they are to participate effectively?
- What rotas are worked? Permanent night staff and part-time staff will need to be considered.

### Finances

- There are costs involved in developing staff.
- Hidden costs of developments/research: doing something a different way may initially slow things down or call for time out from clinical areas for meetings etc.
- Returns may be slow in coming: practice may not immediately change and therefore return on investments may not be immediate.

- What is the cost of employing PDNs, especially since their contribution is less tangible than that of clinically based staff?

### Staff need

- What's in it for me? Staff will need to understand the relevance to themselves as well as to patient care and professional issues.
- Will staff have to undertake work in their own time or will the trust support them to do it in work time?
- What support will staff get (e.g. clinical supervision)?
- Are there hidden management agendas? (If I'm not involved, will I be sacked?)

### Management support

- Does the trust board support the PDN post? Are they and other managers aware that probably the most the organisation can expect after a year is the laying of the foundations and perhaps a framework for practice development and research?
- How are managers selling the posts? Do they see them as a threat / an inconvenience / an asset / something that can be dropped in times of financial difficulty / a quick fix for all ills?
- Will they utilise the post-holders to drive forward genuine developments or use them for hidden agendas such as damming poor practice, or dealing with operational issues such as skill-mix reviews and accountability issues?

### Accountability

- Advisory roles can be seen as just that: 'I don't have to take your advice if it doesn't suit me or I don't like what I'm hearing.'
- When developments occur, who will be accountable? How does the PDN create a safe environment for developments to take place?
- Will practitioners be happy, in terms of accountability and responsibility, with any changes to practice?

### Model used

- Discussed previously. Anecdotal evidence, however, suggests that a strategic approach is more effective.
- How will practice development nurses work with other staff (e.g. allied health professionals and clinical nurse specialists)?
- How will medical support be extracted?

### Evaluation strategies

- How will the effectiveness of the posts be measured?

## CONCLUSION

This chapter has focused purely on practice development as a discreet entity with dedicated practice development roles. I have deliberately not included all the other new roles that have developed over the years, such as clinical nurse specialists, nurse practitioners, and the like, since they are more focused on direct patient outcomes and changing the face of the profession. That is not to say that they do not have a contribution to make. As previously mentioned, all aspects of practice development at all levels are interlinked.

For the role of the PDN, much will depend on where the post is placed within the organisation or the current economic climate. Practice development (and the post-holder) is often viewed as a luxury in times of cash crisis. Additionally, there is potential for conflict within the role. This will be explored later in the book, but it is important to acknowledge that what the organisation expects of the post-holder may not necessarily be in congruence with the staff's expectations.

I am sorry that I have been unable to give you the definitive answer to the question that the chapter poses. But that is the fun of practice development. It can't be categorised but it is rewarding. Even if it does take four hours to explain what you do.

---

**Key points ▶**

- Practice development and professional development are inexorably linked, but do have separate and distinct elements.
- A variety of models can be used to facilitate practice development within an organisation.
- At present, there are no nationally agreed clinical or academic qualifications required of a practice development nurse

---

**RECOMMENDED READING**

Redfern, S., Normand, C., Christian, S., Gilmore, A., Murrells, T., Norman, I. and Stevens, W. (1997) An evaluation of Nursing Development Units, *NT Research* 2(4), 292–303.

Unsworth, J. (2000) Practice development: a concept analysis. *Journal of Nursing Management*, 8, 317–326.

---

**REFERENCES**

Christian, S. and Norman, I. (1998) Clinical leadership in nursing development units. *Journal of Advanced Nursing* 27, 108–116.

Department of Health (2001) *Essence of Care: Patient–Focused Benchmarking for Health Care Practitioners*. London.

Garbett, R. and McCormack, B. (2001) The experience of practice development: an exploratory telephone interview study. *Journal of Clinical Nursing* 10, 94–102.

Gerrish, K. and Ferguson, A. (2000) Nursing development units: factors influencing their progress. *British Journal of Nursing* 9(10), 626–630.

Kitson, A. (1994) *Clinical Nursing Practice Development and Research Activity in the Oxford Region*. Centre for Practice Development and Research, National Institute for Nursing, Oxford.

Mallett, J., Cathmoir, D., Hughes, P. and Whitby, E. (1997). Forging new roles. *Nursing Times* 93(18), 38–39.

Pearson, A. (1983) *The Clinical Nursing Unit*. Heinemann, London.

Redfern, S. and Murrells, T. (1998) Research, audit and networking activity in nursing development units. *NT Research* 3(4), 275–287.

Redfern, S., Normand, C., Christian, S., Gilmore, A., Murrells, T., Norman, I. and

Stevens, W. (1997) An evaluation of Nursing Development Units, *NT Research* 2(4), 292–303.

United Kingdom Central Council for Nursing, Midwifery and Health Visiting (1992) *The Scope of Professional Practice*. London.

Unsworth, J. (2000) Practice development: a concept analysis. *Journal of Nursing Management* 8, 317–326.

Wright, S. (1989) Defining the Nursing Development Unit. *Nursing Standard* 4(7), 29–31.

---

Practice Development Forum – contact the Foundation of Nursing

Foundation of Nursing Studies
32 Buckingham Palace Road, London SW1W 0RE
Tel: 020 7233 5750
Fax: 020 7233 5759
Email: admin@fons.org
http://www.fons.org/

RCN Research and Development Coordinating Centre – Practice Development (UK-wide)
http://www.man.ac.uk/rcn/ukwide/ukpracdev.html

The Centre for the Development of Nursing Policy and Practice
Baines Wing, University of Leeds, Leeds LS2 9UT
Tel: 0113 233 1300
Email: l.j.yates@leeds.ac.uk
http://www.leeds.ac.uk/healthcare/centre/progs/npd.html

Nottingham School of Nursing – Practice Development and Research Centre
http://www.nott.ac.uk/nursing/research/nurse.html

Nursing and Midwifery Practice Development Unit (nmpdu)
Elliott House, 8–10 Hillside Crescent, Edinburgh EH7 5EA
Tel: 0131 623 4287
Fax: 0131 623 4299
Email: info@nmpdu.org
http://www.nmpdu.org/

# 3 DEVELOPING A STRATEGY FOR IMPLEMENTING PRACTICE DEVELOPMENT

*Rob McSherry*

## INTRODUCTION

The term 'practice development' (PD) is gaining monumental recognition for its value in supporting individual health care professionals, teams, and organisations in meeting the challenges of a modernising National Health Service (NHS) in the quest to provide continuous quality improvements and excellence in practice. To demonstrate and maintain excellence in practice requires team-working, interdisciplinary collaboration, effective communication, internal and external partnerships, and a willingness to learn and share with and from each other, including users of the NHS. To contribute to effective individual, team and organisation, PD requires support, investment, and, most importantly, recognition from health care professionals themselves. Recognition that practice development is an integral part of all of our roles and that it is everyone's responsibility to advance and evaluate practice. The challenge facing individual health care professionals, teams, and organisations is how to start advancing or evaluating practice in a busy, stressful, and time-conscious environment like the NHS. The key to resolving these and other obstacles for individuals, teams, and organisations is to 'recognise the complexity of the clinical environment if they want to effect change and tailor any developments to suit local context' (Page, 2001, 36). The difficulty for many health care professionals is in identifying: Where am I now? Where do I start and how do I create a baseline so that improvements or a decline in the standards of individual, team, or organisational practice can be demonstrated?

Taking the above into consideration this chapter explores how practice development can be used to enhance individual, team, and organisational quality. This is achieved firstly by describing the relationship between PD and quality: how individual health care professionals with or without a remit of PD in their job description can utilise PD in support of continued professional development (CPD) and the quest for lifelong learning and evidence-based practice. This is illustrated by referring to Individual Personal/Professional Development Plans, clinical supervision, action learning sets, networking, sharing, and disseminating practice. Secondly, the chapter examines how individuals, teams, and organisations can create and undertake baseline measurement of new or existing practices by focusing on audit, comparative benchmarking, organisational standards, and accreditation. Thirdly, a case study highlights how the author previously used a five-stage 'practice review template' to establish existing practices having just commenced a new job. This consisted of designing and establishing the standards for measurement, assessing practices against the set template, an analysis of the results, and dissemination of findings. This was followed by an evaluation after implementation of the recommendations.

## MEASURING AND EVALUATING PRACTICE: THE RELATIONSHIP BETWEEN PRACTICE DEVELOPMENT AND QUALITY ASSURANCE

Pearson *et al.* (1987) indicates that after Donabedian's introduction of the 'structure, process, and outcome' model for assessing, implementing, and evaluating the effectiveness of clinical practices, many new models have emerged, all of which continue to measure the complexities of practices in the ever-changing, challenging, and expanding clinical environment of the National Health Service and other health and social settings.

No one would dispute the notion that quality assurance is essential in ensuring the 'changing of poor practice into good practice'. Neither would anyone dispute that the measuring and judging of such things as standards in isolation is of little use if the service organisation providing the service to patients remains unchanged as a result of the standards. Standards in this chapter are defined as a level that others accept as the baseline for good practice, or the desired level of achievement (Schroeder and Maibusch, 1984).

The Department of Health (DoH) White Papers *The New NHS: Modern and Dependable* (DoH, 1997) and *A First Class Service: Quality in the New NHS* (DoH, 1998a) emphasise the importance of improving and assuring the quality of care, treatment, and services through principles of clinical governance. Clinical governance is the key framework for guaranteeing quality to the public and the NHS in ensuring that practices whether these be clinical, managerial, or educational are based upon the research evidence (McSherry and Haddock, 1999).

According to the White Papers it would appear that quality improvements have now been placed at the forefront of the NHS agenda and clinical effectiveness as well as cost effectiveness is to be evaluated and measured against national indicators of success. The new structures and systems proposed are:

- a set of National Service Frameworks (NSFs), developed with nationally agreed standards, covering major care areas and disease groups such as cancer services, heart disease, and mental health and illness;
- a new performance framework created with a scorecard of quality in which effectiveness and efficiency measures, rather than the previous cost and activity focus, will be used to measure performance of individual health authorities, NHS trusts, and, potentially, individual health care professionals (this framework may be used in future league tables);
- the National Institute for Clinical Excellence (NICE), responsible for

the assessment of new technologies and producing guidelines for the NHS;

- the Commission for Health Improvement (CHI), to monitor the quality of clinical services at local level and intervene if necessary to deal with problems.

A new system of 'clinical governance' was introduced which is able to demonstrate in both primary and secondary care that systems are in place which guarantee clinical quality improvements at all levels of health care provision. Health care organisations will be explicitly accountable for the quality of services they provide, with the Chief Executive carrying ultimate responsibility, just as they do for financial management. The CHI will ensure that health care organisations fulfil their responsibilities for clinical governance.

In clinical governance, support for, and application of, evidence-based practice is a key feature. Evidence-based practice provides health professionals with the confidence that their interventions, clinical or managerial, are informed by a current and appropriate knowledge base, and ensures the necessary skills are acquired. Practice and guidelines can then be audited and measured against agreed standards (local or national).

Practice development is an ideal vehicle to realise the potential of clinical governance but goes unmentioned in much of the literature. The fundamental aim of PD is 'to act in partnership, providing support between clinical practice, education and management, enabling them to increase research utilisation' (Bassett, 1995; see also Cutcliffe and Bassett, 1997). Taking this into account, practice development provides a foundation for individuals, teams, and organisations to utilise in the quest for quality because it addresses the identification and management of risks, the auditing of standards/practices, the continued professional development of staff, and the sharing and dissemination of practices. Essentially this type of approach to PD promotes evidence-based practice through the integration of clinical expertise with the best available external evidence from systematic research (Sackett *et al.*, 1997) following an evaluation of existing or newly devised standards for practice. It could be argued that practice development is ideal for promoting best practice within the context of clinical governance because it is pertinent to all health and social care professionals, teams, and organisations. Despite there being an enormous amount of literature available on quality assurance, standards, and the use of measurement tools to evaluate patient/user satisfaction and patient/user care, many NHS trusts and health and social care establishments continue to encounter obstacles preventing their organisation from using the instruments. See Box 3.1

Practice development advisors or individuals with a remit to facilitate practice development or innovations in practice provide individuals, teams, and organisations with an opportunity to resolve the obstacles identified in Box 3.1 to measuring and evaluating existing or new

*Box 3.1*

Obstacles preventing the development and utilisation of measurement instrument/tools to evaluate practice

*Selection difficulties*

- How to access the information?
- What is the best tool to use?
- How to implement the tool?
- The difficulty of choosing an indicator tool that meets the requirements of the service.

*Practice constraints*

- Lack of the time needed to complete and interpret the apparatus.
- The difficulty in ensuring accuracy and consisting in data recording.
- The costs incurred by bringing in outside agencies to perform reviews of practice.

*Interpretation/evaluation difficulties*

- What to do with the data when available.
- Inability to implement the findings once the results are available.

practices. This is because in many instances the roles and responsibilities of a practice development advisor are aligned to evaluating changes in practice. The difficulty facing some health and social care professionals and individuals with a designated remit to facilitate practice development is in prioritising and establishing a strategy for their own personal and professional development.

## PRACTICE DEVELOPMENT: THE IMPORTANCE OF ESTABLISHING A STRATEGY FOR INDIVIDUAL PERSONAL AND PROFESSIONAL DEVELOPMENT

As outlined in Chapter 2, the diversity, complexity, and range of roles and responsibilities expected of individuals and teams with a remit for developing or evaluating practice are vast and varied. This could be explained by the fact that each health or social care organisation, team, or individual is unique, having different and preferred working cultures, environments, and management and leadership styles. These factors make each occasion for practice development unique because it is about individuals or teams rising to the challenges imposed by the complexity and diversity of different organisational cultures, clinical environments, workforce pressures, and the support shown by leaders and management within the organisation. Practice development provides hope and opportunity in health and social settings because it is about making small changes in response to local priorities and needs (Wills, 2000). The challenge facing some health care professionals and those with a remit to facilitate practice development is in identifying and prioritising their own needs. This is a highly important and often neglected aspect of practice development and continued professional development. The failure of individuals with a remit to facilitate practice development to focus on their own continued professional development seems to occur predominately because practice development is about facilitating *others* to innovate or evaluate practices through the establishment of partnerships, multi-professional collaboration, effective communication, and the sharing of practices and so the individual fails to focus on their *own* personal/professional needs.

## Activity 3.1

Having looked at your job description, note down what you see as the individual attributes and skills required to undertake the role and responsibilities of practice development. How do you plan to achieve these attributes and skills?

For more information read on and compare your findings with those outlined in the chapter.

Having undertaken Activity 3.1, you will appreciate how diverse the demands of the PD role are and how difficult it is to quantify them. Perhaps this is why when one is challenged to summarise what you do, it is difficult to do so without justifying all the attributes the post entails. From my personal experiences working in practice development and from reading and reviewing some of the literature, the post of practice development can be viewed in three ways: individual personal attributes, essential skills, and individual development and support.

### Practice development: the importance of individual personal attributes

To undertake the role of practice development successfully it would appear that six key themes emerge as essential individual personal attributes. See Box 3.2.

**Box 3.2**

Practice development: the importance of individual personal attributes.

- Motivate
- Facilitate
- Innovate
- Inform
- Encourage
- Support

NB. This is not an exhaustive list and the points are not in any order of priority.

Practice development is about *encouraging* and *motivating* staff to *innovate* or *evaluate* practices in the quest for improved quality. To achieve this successfully, practice development requires individuals and teams who are *informed* of the various components of clinical governance – risk management, audit, research and development, so that the appropriate *support* and *guidance* can be afforded to the individual, team, and organisation.

## Essential qualities for successful practice development

The essential qualities to be successful in practice development are listed in Box 3.3.

---

**Box 3.3**

Essential qualities for successful practice development.

- Commitment
- Respect
- Experience
- Approachable
- An agent of change
- Supportive
- Good listener

NB. This is not an exhaustive list and the points are not in any order of priority.

---

Arguably, one might say that all health and social care professionals have or should have the qualities outlined in Box 3.3. However, in practice development these qualities become even more important when one is facilitating the development or evaluation of new or existing ways of working. The individuals, team, organisation, and the practice development facilitator require *commitment* to harnessing and maintaining colleague enthusiasm to tackle the issues involved in advancing practice. Listening, empowering, valuing, and involving the respective colleagues/users with the innovation can enhance changes in practice. This approach to practice development affords *respect* from the facilitator towards their colleagues, an essential skill that is often neglected in practice development.

Successful practice development initiatives depend upon the *experience* and *approachability* of the facilitator in encouraging, supporting, and, where applicable, resourcing innovations in practice. The facilitator can become a *change agent* by providing an objective, non-judgmental, open, honest approach to practice development. Successful practice development in my experience requires the utilisation and integration of personal attributes and essential skills such that the facilitation and empowerment of individuals, teams, and organisations is based upon promoting teamwork and multi-professional collaboration via effective communication. The challenge for some health and social care professionals with or without a remit for practice development is in identifying and prioritising their own individual and professional requirements and the support needed to facilitate and manage change. It would appear that many health care professionals and teams with a remit for practice development direct their attentions so effectively to the organisation's and their professional colleagues' objectives that they jeopardise their own CPD and support networks. To sustain and facilitate practice change, regardless of its nature and magnitude, over the long term requires support. Support for individuals facilitating changes in practice could be enhanced by ensuring that some or all of the following become an integral part of the practice development role: an Individual Personal/Professional Development Plan, clinical supervision, action learning sets, networking, sharing and disseminating practice.

### Individual Personal/Professional Development Plans

As outlined in Chapter 2, the role, responsibilities, and models promoting practice development in health and social care are vast, varied, and often unique to the organisation's culture, management, and environment (Page, 2001). Likewise practice development seems to mean different things to different health and social care professionals and professional disciplines. This is borne out by discussions with health care professionals with a remit for practice development and by reviewing job descriptions over the past couple of years. What seems to emerge is the diversity of roles, responsibilities, and expectations of the post-holder. Some posts have a single remit for PD whereas others have a partnership role for facilitating PD along with the management of other important organisational systems and processes such as risk management, quality, clinical audit, or education and training. Recently, many PD posts have been redeveloped to facilitate and accommodate the clinical governance and evidence-based practice agenda. It is this variation in roles and expectations that makes PD so interesting and rewarding for the post-holder and teams. The difficulties and dilemma it creates at times are in prioritising what should be addressed first and in working out how to accommodate two employers, especially when you have a post based on a partnership arrangement.

A way forward to resolving these and other issues associated with such a diverse and unique post is to ensure that you have a firm and clear understanding of what your job description entails along with an understanding of what your employer expects from you. A strategy of how you intend to assess, implement, and evaluate achievement of the key roles and responsibilities should be your number one priority. This can be made more successful by linking this to your own continued professional development and Individual Personal Review (IPR) and Personal and Professional Development Plan (PDP).

### Continued practice and professional development

The term 'CPD' was originally mentioned in White Papers (DoH, 1997; 1998a, b) where the government set out its long-term goal of modernising the NHS, with the key focus for change centred on quality improvements. Continued professional development is defined as 'A process of lifelong learning for all individuals and teams which meets the needs of patients and delivers the health outcomes and health care priorities of the NHS and which enables professionals to expand and fulfil their potential' (NHS Executive, 1998, 42). To ensure that an organisation and staff deliver a high quality service, they need to have sound knowledge and well-developed competencies to perform their roles efficiently and effectively. Lifelong learning and CPD should be seen as an ongoing process in ensuring that practices are the most effective and up to date. From my experience in practice development, CPD is a highly important element for the success in the role. It is important at an individual level in ensuring that you maintain and enhance your own essential skills and attributes. This will enable you to fulfil the role successfully as well as provide a means of accessing and supporting other individuals and teams in advancing or evaluating new or existing practice. To achieve life long learning, health care organisations must have robust systems and processes to ensuring CPD for their entire body of employees.

In practice development it is imperative to encourage all staff to agree that CPD is the beginning of a process concerned with developing a culture of lifelong learning – a culture that if successfully created could become the basis for sound and lasting advances in practice. To support practice development within the CPD framework requires a robust system and process for the delivery of CPD with local ownership. In practice development this approach to supporting innovation should be viewed as a long-term objective and could take several years to achieve. This is why it requires backing from the Chairs and Chief Executives of health care organisations. They have a key role to play in ensuring CPD via collaboration and communication between managers, human resources departments, and nursing and medical education committees and in ensuring that the educational aspect of CPD meets their organisations' and professional staff's requirements.

Practice development can help you facilitate the development of a system for CPD in a health care organisation, trust, directorate, team or for individuals. To do this effectively it is imperative to implement the points outlined in the Health Services Circular (HSC) 1999/154, *Continuing Professional Development: Quality in the New NHS* (National Health Service Executive, 1999). To illustrate how this can be achieved, the following example is adapted from Pearce and McSherry (2000) with kind permission from Blackwell Science Publishers.

## Practice development: facilitating the implementing of continuing professional development at an individual and organisation level

The HSC 1999/154 encourages organisations in the NHS to adopt a focused approach to ensuring the delivery of high quality care – an approach that could be enhanced by the development of robust CPD. In applying this principle the concept of management by objectives could be introduced. This style of managing CPD enables the trust to anticipate and highlight important issues relevant to the needs of their health care population. Corporate objectives are set before the start of the financial year which are specific to the core elements of the trust's business plan. From these core objectives, sub-objectives for clinical and general mangers are established and linked to the Personal Development Plans for their staff. Personal Development Plans are linked to individuals' annual performance appraisal, where the employee and manager review the year's progress and assess strengths, weaknesses, opportunities, and threats (SWOT analysis), jointly agreeing an individual plan for the next 12 months with a six-monthly review. This approach enables the trust to systematically identify the important national, regional, and local issues to inform a coherent and coordinated strategy in achieving its objectives. This approach to CPD ensures that the trust is working collaboratively as a team. Figure 3.1 illustrates a model for the CPD processes.

This approach to enhancing quality is ideal for supporting practice development because the new innovations or ways of evaluating new and existing practices could be directly linked to the objectives of the organisation, directorate, team, or individual's performance. Likewise it is worth noting here that CPD is a key element of the Investors in People Award that many health care organisations and teams aspire to

**Figure 3.1**

A model to aid the integration of CPD into health care organisation

| Phase I | February/March |
| --- | --- |
| Corporate objectives assigned to Executive Directors | |

| Phase 2 | April |
| --- | --- |
| Executive and General Clinical Managers agree objectives to address corporate objectives | |

| Phase 3 | April |
| --- | --- |
| General and Clinical Managers and Head of Departments agree their respective departments' objectives<br>PDPs agreed | |

| Phase 4 | April |
| --- | --- |
| Employees and Head of Departments agree individual objectives | |

achieve in demonstrating their support of staff. (For more information on this award, visit http:www.iipuk.co.uk.) It is evident from the above information that CPD and lifelong learning are integral aspects of practice development and can only be achieved by mutual collaboration, respect, openness, and honesty between employees and employers about how the individual and organisation are performing. Successful implementation depends on adequate research and genuine commitment and support from all parties involved.

The difficulties for some health and social care professionals with a remit for advancing practice as part of their IPR or professional development is in establishing and maintaining sound supporting structures for themselves or their teams. In practicedevelopment clinical supervision could help overcome many of the practical issues associated with setting and maintaining the right level of support.

## CLINICAL SUPERVISION

Clinical supervision is defined as 'a formal arrangement that enables nurses, midwives and health visitors to discuss their work regularly with another experienced professional. Clinical supervision involves reflecting on practice in order to learn from experience and improve confidence' (Kohner, 1994). Clinical supervision is described as a formal process of professional support and learning, enabling individual practitioners to develop knowledge and competence, assume responsibility for their own practice, and enhance consumer protection and safety of care in complex situations. It is central to the process of learning and to the scope of professional practice and should be seen as a means of encouraging self-assessment and analytical and reflective skills (DoH, 1993).

After reflecting upon the above definitions and descriptions of clinical supervision, it is easy to see why it has the potential to support individuals, teams, and organisations who wish to advance or evaluate practice, since the core principles behind clinical supervision focus on:

- safeguarding standards
- promoting professional development and expertise
- delivering and evaluating the quality care (Kohner, 1994).

These are all key elements for an individual or a model of practice development. The challenge for individuals, teams, and organisations is in utilising a model of clinical supervision to form an informal yet supportive framework for advancing or evaluating practice. Bassett (1999) provides an excellent guide to implementing clinical supervision, which addresses the challenges by drawing upon a variety of experts from clinical and practice development settings. Bassett's text provides an opportunistic framework for implementing and evaluating practice and also outlines the advantages and disadvantages of using such a method of providing support for individuals, teams, or an organisation. If clinical supervision is not possible then alternative forms of supporting practice development are by means of action learning and learning sets.

## ACTION LEARNING AND LEARNING SETS

Action learning (AL) is defined as a 'continuous process of learning and reflection, supported by colleagues, with the intention of getting things done' (McGill and Beaty, 1995). This is achieved by bringing individuals together in a small group known as a 'learning set' where set members' ideas can be challenged in a supportive non-threatening environment with the support and guidance of a set facilitator. Action learning is different to traditional ways of teaching and learning because it focuses on the individual's current, not past, experience and situation, requiring active involvement in resolving real, not historic, case studies. See Figure 3.2.

Action learning is an ideal way to support individuals with a remit for practice development because, as a set member, they will be able to discuss ideas and issues associated with their role and responsibilities and be supported in a structured way to advance practice. Likewise, to undertake training to become a facilitator of AL is an ideal way of:

- advancing practice in a team and organisation
- encouraging and assuring effective collaboration and communication
- providing support in a informal non-threatening structured way networking
- sharing and disseminating practice.

The advantages of AL to health and social care and professionals with or without a remit for practice development can be categorised as follows. The process:

- empowers participants by encouraging them to take charge of their own problems/issues;

*Figure 3.2*

| Traditional learning | Action Learning |
|---|---|
| Historic case studies | Current case studies |
| Individual orientation | Group-based learning |
| Learning about others | Learning about self and others |
| Studying other organisations | Studying own organisation |
| Programmed knowledge | Questions plus programmed knowledge |
| Planning | Planning and doing |
| Arm's Length | Arm in arm with clients |
| Input based | Output/result based |
| Past oriented | Present and future oriented |
| Low risk | Higher risk |
| Passive | Active |

- encourages skills of problem solving;
- accommodates a wide variety of situations because of its flexibility in design;
- increases transfer of learning.

The weaknesses of AL are demonstrating its actual value to indivi-duals, team, or organisational performances because of the flexibility in its method and diversity in accommodating the uniqueness of each learning set and its participants. Although it remains difficult to measure and quantify AL, from my experiences of using it in health care practice and education, the impact on individual personal learning and devel-opment is vast. The difficulty for some health care professionals and organisations is in sharing and disseminating experiences at a local, regional, or international level. This remains a challenge for some individuals, teams, and organisations.

## NETWORKING: SHARING AND DISSEMINATING PRACTICE

It would be fair to say that there are many and varied ways of sharing and disseminating developments or evaluations of new or existing practices (Fig 3.3) Some have been successful in efficiently and effec-tively promoting quality; some have not. In practice development it is essential that a cultural and clinical environment based on mutual learning and sharing is nurtured. Without fostering this approach to developing practice, how can any individual, team, or organisation promote quality care, treatments, interventions, or services? Regardless of the nature of the innovation or evaluation of practice, the notion of sharing and disseminating the findings, the evaluation of the innovation provided, and how the process enabled the change to occur should all be seen as an integral part of practice development. How can the NHS expect to modernise if the health and social care professionals working within it themselves fail to share with and learn from each other?

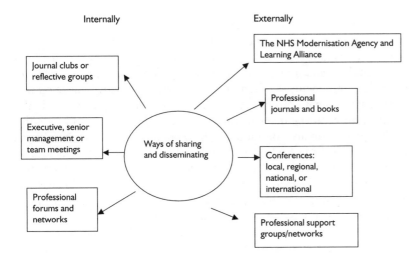

**Figure 3.3**

Ways of sharing and disseminating practice

Successful practice development not only requires individuals with a remit to facilitate practice development but the creation of a culture and working environment, and teams within it, that promote and maintain a philosophy of multi-professional collaboration. If this is to be taken seriously in the future, multi-professional partnerships or collaborations must become more than a throw-away phrase and should be recognised as the working, sharing, and disseminating of practice *together*. The obstacles hindering some individuals and teams from sharing innovations or evaluations in practice are based on a lack of confidence, support, or resources to do so. As health care professionals, we tend to feel that what we have done is not good enough to publish or present at a conference when quite the opposite could be said.

To resolve these feelings and break down the barriers to sharing and dissemination it is imperative to seek the support of other departments, organisations, or professionals to help you individually or as a team. At a local internal level, departments such as information technology, clinical audit, research and development, or clinical governance may be able to offer some practical advice and guidance. They may also provide resources or financial support to facilitate presentation and the best ways of sharing and disseminating your findings. Alternatively, you could liase externally with the modernisation agency www.nhs.uk/modernnhs, whose remit is to endorse the principles of clinical governance by encouraging up-to-date multi-professional collaborative working and the sharing of practice through a variety of working collaborations such as primary care and coronary heart disease. Similarly contacting higher education, research departments, personal tutors or academics, article editors or publishers directly to aid you should be considered. Sometimes the dilemma is not how to contact and ask for advice or support but how to find the best way to communicate your developments in practice. McSherry *et al.* (2002) offer practical steps in this area by focusing your attention on issues such as target audiences, presentation styles and skills, resourcing, and how to facilitate change.

In summary it could be argued that as a part of professional accountability and the modernisation agenda all health and social care professionals should be responsible for practice development. This would be difficult to dispute. Successful practice development requires individuals, teams, and organisations that proactively foster a culture based on principles of openness, honesty, and trust. Practice development requires investment both in those individuals with a remit for facilitating it and in all health and social care professionals, who should be continually professionally developing throughout their careers. Given adequate resourcing and investment, individuals or teams facilitating practice development need to be able to demonstrate the impacts they are having on performance. 'Performance management' in this instance refers to demonstrating how practices have or have not had an impact on patient outcomes, in enhancing efficiency and effectiveness of services, or in promoting quality improvements. The challenge for some health care professionals or teams with a remit for advancing practice is: once you have established your supporting systems and structures, how do you proceed to demonstrate the benefits of the post or team to other individuals, teams, or the organisation?

## DEVELOPING AND IMPLEMENTING A STRATEGY TO MEASURE AND EVALUATE THE IMPACT OF PRACTICE DEVELOPMENT AT A TEAM OR ORGANISATION LEVEL

As mentioned in Chapter 2, the diversity in the roles, responsibilities, and expectations of practice development is often as complex and difficult to describe as the organisational models. This phenomenon can be easily explained by the fact that each health care organisation is unique in its culture and management and the way it values and supports advances in practice and, more importantly, its staff. This diversity in culture and management creates a dilemma for individuals and teams working in practice development when trying to measure the impact their role or team has had in promoting continuous quality among individuals, teams, and the organisation. To resolve this dilemma in measuring and evaluating the potential advantages and disadvantages of practice development at an individual, team, or organisational level, the individual or team needs to adopt a creative and flexible approach using a variety of methods, departments, and resources. To demonstrate the efficiency and effectiveness of a practice development post or team requires the individual or team to have the necessary knowledge and skills to measure and evaluate quality. The commencement of this process of evaluation should coincide with the commencement of the role by undertaking a baseline measurement of existing practices.

## Activity 3.2 ——————————————————————————

Note down as many methods as you can think of that might aid you in measuring and evaluating practices.

For more information read on and compare your notes with the remainder of this section.

Having undertaken Activity 3.2, you will appreciate that there are a variety of ways measuring and evaluating practice: clinical audit, patient satisfaction surveys, formal research with randomised control trials, action research, leadership and management style assessment tools, and change models, to name but a few. To try to explain the advantages and disadvantages of the various methods of measuring and evaluating practice would be unwise. What is worth pointing out at this stage is that the key thing is to apply those approaches that best suit the area of practice. For example, if an area of practice development involves a clinical team seeking the views of users for a given service, a patient satisfaction survey or research focus group could be used, either alone or combined. Essentially, evaluating practice is about utilising the appropriate measurement or evaluative templates at the right time.

To help you develop your knowledge and skills in measuring and evaluating practice this section of the chapter will now focus on describing three current ways to evaluate practice: audit, comparative benchmarking, and organisational standards and accreditation.

### Audit: an ally not a threat to practice development

In practice development some health care professionals always associate audit with medical interventions because of the association with the term 'clinical audit'. Clinical audit is viewed as a systematic, formal way in which to measure and improve the quality of care. In general, clinical audit has predominantly focused on one professional group, e.g. nurses; care plan audits or multidisciplinary audits. More recently, multi-professional audits are occurring which are performed by a mixed group of health and social care professionals as seen in auditing the outcome of stroke care.

To measure and evaluate new or existing ways of working within a practice development framework the use of 'multi-professional audit' is the only way forward. This is because many advances in or evaluations of new or existing practices are based on multi-professional collaborations and team-working in which it is difficult to isolate an individual's contributions to quality enhancements. Multidisciplinary audit in practice development 'involves systematically looking at procedures used for diagnosis, care and treatment, examining how associated resources are used and investigating the effect care has on the outcome and quality of life for the patient' (DoH, 1993).

The main points of this definition are that multi-professional audit must be systematic and critical. The critical analysis should be used as a constructive mechanism to improve quality and demonstrate the outcomes for the patient, user, or service. Audit can be used to evaluate the efficiency and effectiveness of any component of practice such as:

- delivery of care, e.g. type of care, place of care, method of delivery;
- timeliness of care, e.g. appropriate time of medication, discharge planning;
- outcomes of care, e.g. complications, changes in function, general health perception, reduction in symptoms. (DoH, 1993)

Multi-professional audit is an ally of practice development because it is about comparing our performance as an individual or team against set standards to demonstrate the effectiveness of the practice provided. This is achieved by the instigation of the audit cycle, as provided by the DoH (1993) and depicted in Figure 3.4, based upon observing, comparing against set standards, implementing change, setting new standards, and again observing and evaluating the benefits of the practice.

In practice development, support is available to help you or teams with instigating the audit process, for example, the Audit Department and access to a set of local, regional, and national standards. This has

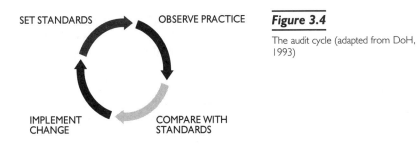

**Figure 3.4**

The audit cycle (adapted from DoH, 1993)

been made easier over the past couple of years by the government's introduction of National Service Frameworks (NSF) and the National Institute for Clinical Excellence (NICE). The introduction of the NSF's and NICE guidelines provides a framework for promoting evidence-based standards and processes for assessing, measuring, and evaluating practice in a multi-professional context. Within practice development it is imperative that you develop your knowledge, skills, and confidence to access and use them.

## Comparative benchmarking: promoting collaborative networking for practice development

Benchmarking is viewed as a 'process of seeking, finding, implementing and sustaining best practice. It is a continuous process of measuring services and practices against other similar areas' (Feely, 2001). This is a useful approach to demonstrating the contributions that practice development makes to teams and organisations by adopting a proactive method for measuring and evaluating new or existing practices. Benchmarking provides an opportunistic, structured approach to promoting best practice by encouraging health and social care professionals, teams, and organisations to share findings about an identified area of care, for example, comparing the levels and standards of record keeping. It is imperative when using benchmarking not to confuse the term with a 'benchmark' in the sense of 'a standard in judging quality, value' (Collins, 1987). A benchmark is the desired standard of performance an individual, team, or organisation is aspiring to reach and is usually identified as a result of benchmarking.

Different types of benchmarking can be undertaken depending upon the practice under review. *Internally*, this is done by comparing similar processes within different sections of the organisation, for example, patient waiting times in different outpatients areas. *Externally*, competitive benchmarking could be used to compare similar size organisations' performance against certain standards, such as on the cost of treatments. *Functional* benchmarking refers to the isolation of functional processes and compares findings such as on non-attendance for outpatients appointments.

The benchmarking process could be seen as cumbersome and time consuming but it is ideal for supporting and evaluating practice. Put simply, the process requires the practitioner to:

- consider the practice requiring a benchmark;
- identify the area of practice to be benchmarked;
- select potential benchmark partners, internally or externally;
- establish data to be captured;
- collect data from both benchmarking partners;
- compare data and determine gaps in performance;
- review processes for deficits;
- communicate finds;
- review targets for future performances;
- adjust targets and develop strategy for improving practice by use of staged, achievable, and realistic goals;
- implement changes with involvement and endorsement of the team;
- review progress after identified period of time (adapted from Feely, 2001).

The brief description identifies the potential advantages of benchmarking for practice development. It encourages a proactive approach to collaborative networking and the sharing of practices. It can be used to encourage multi-professional team-working, especially in areas of practice that require input from a variety of professional disciplines, e.g. rehabilitation.

The disadvantages of using benchmarking seem to be associated with time commitments and releasing staff to undertake the benchmarking. Practices where possible should be compared and contrasted in promoting and developing best practices. Benchmarking provides such a mechanism for all health care professionals and disciplines to use in the future. Some references to benchmarks can be found on the following useful websites:

- Benchmarking:  http://nmap.ac.uk/text/browse/mesh/detail/C0525063 L0743225.html
- University of Central Lancashire Paediatric Benchmarking: http://www.uclan.ac.uk/facs/health/bench/benchbac.htm
- The Benchmarking Centre: http://www.benchmarking.co.uk

### Organisational standards and accreditation

Over the past 15 years the development of organisational standards and accreditation of clinical excellence have emerged as challenges and aspirations for teams and organisations in demonstrating best practice against a rigorous set of criteria or standards. Initially, Nursing Development Units (NDU) (Lathlean, 1997) followed by Practice Development Units (PDU) (Page, 1998) emerged as the forerunners for teams and organisations to use in demonstrating a culture based on organisational and management leadership – leadership that is founded on a philosophy of promoting excellence in team-working, multi-professional collaboration or partnerships by encouraging staff to use research to advance and evaluate their practice.

In the contemporary NHS many organisational standards and accreditation frameworks continue to emerge to assist health care professionals, teams, and organisations in demonstrating an achieved level of quality for a given service. The Commission for Health Improvements (CHI), European Foundation Quality Management (EFQM), Investors in People (IIP), Practice/Nurse Development Unit Accreditation, Clinical Negligence Scheme for Trust (CNST), and Charter Mark are to name but a few. The potential benefits of each of these frameworks lie in offering a set of criteria for measuring a given practice to a set standard or level of excellence. For example, IIP relates to assessing organisational support and staff development. The Commission for Health Improvements reviews how a health care organisation is meeting the challenge of implementing clinical governance. The two are different, yet equally valuable to advancing and evaluating practice. The major problems of organisational standards and accreditation in the NHS today are in the duplication of time, resourcing, and support needed by individuals, teams, and organisations in collecting, collating and providing the evidence in demonstrating the acquired standards. Health care organisations seem to be pressurised to meet not just the criteria for one award but for several at any one time. Organisational standards and accreditation are essential for demonstrating acquired levels of excellence in the NHS. They provide excellent frameworks for promoting quality improvements and as a result support practice development. However, from my recent experiences of working with organisational standards in practice, along with assessing levels of achieved practice, they require organisational and management support, resourcing, and financial backing.

What seems to be missing to aid practice development is any unifying and linking of these various frameworks. For example, if you go for the award of PDU/NDU and provide robust evidence to achieve the standards for valuing staff and their development, surely this evidence could be used to support similar standards within the IIP. According to McSherry and Kell (2002), it appears today that six core areas of practice have emerged that relate to most organisational and accreditation packages in health and social care. These should also form the basis for advancing and evaluating practice:

- working in organisations
- collaborative working
- user-focused care
- continuous quality improvements
- performance management
- measuring efficiency and effectiveness.

(for more information, see Box 3.4)

Although the above core standards appear broad, many substandards are available to support the achievement of the standard. For example, to demonstrate the achievement of the standard working in organisations evidence would need to be provided that illustrates how the management support was provided which endorses innovation via open channels of communication in encouraging and empowering staff to share ideas. Practice development is about focusing individuals, teams, and organisations to create a culture in which clinical or practice excellence can occur. By focusing on the six core standards identified above, practices at an individual, team, and organisational level can be measured and evaluated.

The difficulty for some individuals, teams, and organisations is in implementing such standards. The final section of this chapter will attempt to demonstrate how this can be possible by providing a case study relating to a baseline assessment of existing practice in a health care organisation via a 'practice review'.

**Box 3.4**

> ### The Excellence in Practice Accreditation Scheme
>
> For more information about the newly developed 'Excellence in Practice' accreditation scheme that enables bench-marking to be undertaken and a level of excellence in practice to be awarded, please contact the University of Teesside, School of Health and Social Care, Middlesbrough, Practice Development team.

## CASE STUDY 3.1

Establishing a baseline: the practice review template

The intention of Case Study 3.1 is to provide you with an example of how practice development can be measured and evaluated by the instigation of a baseline assessment. As mentioned in Chapter 2, practice development is difficult to describe because each organisational management culture is unique. Likewise when referring to the practice review it is important to take organisational, environmental and cultural factors into account.

### WHY THE PRACTICE REVIEW TEMPLATE WAS DEVELOPED

Because of the challenges created by the recent government reforms purported by the White Papers (DoH, 1997; 1998a, b) and the Patient's Charter (1992), many providers of health and social care need to re-examine ways in which communication and developments of quality standards can be achieved in their setting. The anticipated rise in activity in acute care services and the reductions in acute beds has placed a growing emphasis on the need to develop a baseline indicator of current clinical practices in order to prepare for the future. The healthcare organisation has certainly prepared for health care in the millennium by undertaking a practice review of the nursing services currently being provided, so that developments can be made in the future.

## DEVISING THE PRACTICE REVIEW

The practice review aims to achieve:

- a baseline indicator of the current standards and quality of nursing and midwifery care in the individual directorates and the organisation;
- provision of a quality and standard measurement tool by ensuring that written criteria are available for the assessment of standards;
- annual use of the measurement tool to evaluate the impact of the education and training provided by the organisation to individual wards, outpatient departments, and directorates throughout the trust;
- provision of a framework for nursing and midwifery education and training in *all* clinical areas;
- detection and facilitation of the sharing of not so good, good, and excellent practices throughout individual wards and directorates;
- implementation of nursing and midwifery development plans in order to enhance the continued improvement of *all* clinical areas.

## METHODS

The development of the template was achieved in five stages: template design, process of delivery, data analysis, presentation of results, and evaluation of progress to date.

## STAGE 1: TEMPLATE DESIGN

The starting point was to establish and agree a criterion to be measured, so that the standards could be observed for compliance. This was achieved after several months of exploring and reviewing literature on the use of the quality and standard measurement tools.

This resulted in the Practice Development Advisers/Lecturers (PDAs) developing their own measurement template, designed to provide a clinical overview of the current practices and availability of resources in the clinical area of nursing and midwifery. It was hoped that, by referring to the team's collective clinical, educational and research experiences, an objective and representative template could be created that would meet the requirements of the clinical areas and the organisation's unique culture, management, and leadership.

The template is directed towards ensuring that current political, educational, professional, and clinical practices are being reviewed, covering the following key areas: care delivery, care planning/documentation, and organisational, educational, corporate, and professional issues in practice, as illustrated in Figure 3.5.

**Figure 3.5**

Example of a practice review
standard

| Directorate | Ward | | Comments | Professional | | | | Comments |
|---|---|---|---|---|---|---|---|---|
| Date ............... | Please tick (✓) box Y/N | | | | | | | |
| CARE DELIVERY | | Y   N | | 29. SCOPE | | | | |
| 1.  System of Care Delivery | Task orientation | ☐  ☐ | | | Y | N | No. | |
| | Team nursing | ☐  ☐ | | IV's | ☐ | ☐ | ☐ | |
| | Complex team nursing | ☐  ☐ | | Venepuncture | ☐ | ☐ | ☐ | |
| | Primary nursing | ☐  ☐ | | Cannulation | ☐ | ☐ | ☐ | |
| | Patient allocation | ☐  ☐ | | Male/female catheterization | ☐ | ☐ | ☐ | |
| | | | | ECG | ☐ | ☐ | ☐ | |
| 2.  Handover | Office report | ☐  ☐ | | NGT | ☐ | ☐ | ☐ | |
| | Office report and introduc- tion bedside | ☐  ☐ | | Defibrillation | ☐ | ☐ | ☐ | |

## STAGE 2: PROCESS OF DELIVERY

The practice review was undertaken by the Practice Development
Advisers with the assistance and cooperation of the Ward/Out Patient
Department Managers and Nurse Specialists. There were six core
standards with 29 individual standards. For example: Philosophy of
Care, System of Care Delivery, Handovers, Documentation, and Scope
of Professional practice.

A total of 49 clinical areas were reviewed throughout seven directorates, as follows: Anaesthetics and Theatres, Maternity and Gynaecology, Mental Health, Surgical, Child Health, Medicine, Orthopaedics,
and Accident and Emergency.

## STAGE 3: DATA ANALYSIS.

The audit template was structured in such a way that a case by variable
matrix was formulated for each of the areas reviewed and entered on to
a spreadsheet for statistical analysis with the aid of SPSS (Statistical
Package for Social Science). The process of transcription is depicted in
Figures 3.6 to 3.8.

Figure 3.6 shows the blank audit form and how it was coded to
resemble the results on Figure 3.7 and how the data finally looked on
the SPSS spreadsheet for data analysis. The case by variable matrix,

| Directorate.................................. | Ward ............................................. |
|---|---|

**CARE DELIVERY**     Please tick box, Y/N

|  |  |  | Y | N |
|---|---|---|---|---|
| I. | System of care delivery | Task allocation | ☐ | ☐ |
|  |  | Team nursing | ☐ | ☐ |
|  |  | Complex team nursing | ☐ | ☐ |
|  |  | Primary nursing | ☐ | ☐ |
|  |  | Patient allocation | ☐ | ☐ |

**Figure 3.6**

Blank template sheet

| DIRECTORATE 5 Medicine |  |  | Yes = I |  |
|---|---|---|---|---|
| Ward        I |  |  | No = 0 |  |
|  |  |  | Y | N |
| I. | System of care | I. Task | 0 | 0 |
|  |  | 2. Team nursing | I | 0 |
|  |  | 3. Complex team nursing | 0 | 0 |
|  |  | 4. Primary nursing | 0 | 0 |
|  |  | 5. Patient allocation | I | 0 |

**Figure 3.7**

Transcription sheet with codes

| CASES | Directorate | System Care I | System Care 2 |
|---|---|---|---|
| I | 5 | 0 | 2 |
| 2 |  |  |  |
| 3 |  |  |  |

**Figure 3.8**

SPSS spreadsheet and variables

Figure 3.8, shows the *cases* in rows – for example, 1 = Blue Ward, 2 = Bill Ward – and *variables* in columns; for example:

Directorate             = 5 = Medicine
System of care delivery 1 = 0 = Task allocation
System of care delivery 2 = 2 = Team nursing

A similar template was devised for review of the care plans.

The above exercise was carried out for 49 different clinical wards/ outpatient departments and covered 29 areas of practice from delivery of care and philosophy of care to organisational policies manuals etc.

## STAGE 4: RESULTS AND DISCUSSION

No statistical analysis was undertaken on the data because there were more variables than cases, which would have resulted in insufficient

**Figure 3.9**

Preferred systems of care delivery

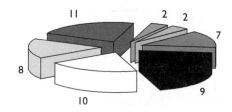

◧ Task Allocation
■ Team Nursing
□ Complex Team Nursing + Management Tasks Allocated to Teams
□ Primary Nursing
▨ Patient Allocation/Case Load
▨ Named Nurse/Clinic
□ Other= A Combined Use of Patient Allocation/Caseload and Named Nurse

numbers for probability testing. The SPSS spreadsheets were used in the production of descriptive frequency and percentile data, along with the production of graphic illustrations. The results provided an overview and baseline of the hospital's current standards of nursing and midwifery clinical, organisational, educational, corporate, and professional practices, set against the standards outlined in the practice review template. Several of the findings are summarised and discussed to provide the reader with an idea of how the final results were presented.

The System of Care Delivery (Standard 1) demonstrated that all 49 areas covered by the practice review had a recognised system of care delivery in operation, as shown in Figure 3.9.

It is encouraging to see that *all* 49 areas covered by the review had a recognised system of care delivery, the benefits of which are well documented in recent nursing literature. For example: improved standards and quality of care, vehicle for delivering nursing process, increased accountability, reduced hospital costs, increased patient and staff satisfaction.

The most commonly used methods of care delivery being practised are: team nursing (19), primary nursing (8), named qualified nurse (2), and caseload (11). If combined the above provides a total of 40 (81.63%), suggesting that a positive approach is being taken to enhance the efficiency and effectiveness of patient care delivery.

## Handovers (Standard 2)

Forty-four of the areas had a method of transferring information, whether clinical or organisational, to other professional colleagues. The most preferred mechanisms are shown in Figure 3.10.

In 89.79% of cases attempts were being made to communicate information to Ward/OPD/Nurse Specialists and other professional colleagues working in the clinical areas. The office report and nurse introduction at the bedside were the most commonly practised methods

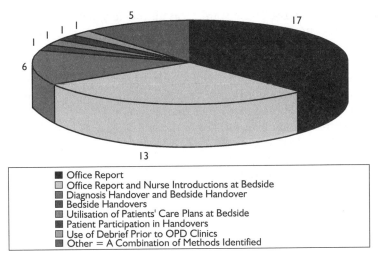

**Figure 3.10**

Handovers

in 55.1% of cases. The time it took for these reports varied between 30 and 60 minutes. Some areas used a combined method of a short office report followed by a bedside handover and utilisation of care plan with patient involvement. A small percentage of outpatient departments were using a debrief to prioritise and give information before the commencement of clinics.

## DOCUMENTATION (STANDARD 3)

Thirty-one areas had a recognised system of recording information. The most preferred methods are shown in Figure 3.11.

Despite 31 (63.26%) areas having a recognised system of recording information, 18 (36.73%) required further work to review their current practices of recording information, in order to ensure that this was done

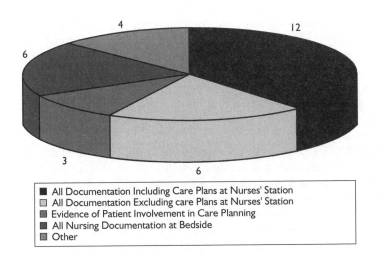

**Figure 3.11**

Documentation

effectively. In most of the ward areas all the documentation was held at the nurses' station, with the exception of care plans, which were held at the bedside. Minimal evidence was available to suggest there was patient/carer involvement in the writing and evaluating of care plans etc. Outpatient departments and Clinical Nurse Specialists tend either to have their own record cards for writing and recording information or to enter information directly into the medical notes.

The strengths and weaknesses of the findings are as follows:

### Strengths

- Systems of care delivery
- Assessment tools
- Clinical audit
- Internal rotation
- Visiting facilities
- Staff development review
- Communication
- Personalising the service
- Resource area
- Link nurses
- Mentorship
- Patient information
- Scope

### Weaknesses

- Handovers
- Documentation/care planning and discharge
- Multidisciplinary collaboration
- Named nurse induction/preceptorship
- Philosophy of care
- Research (evidence-based care)

The practice review certainly showed that steps are being taken to ensure that patients/relatives are communicated with and catered for in a variety of ways. For example, visiting facilities, personalising the service, patient information, and resource areas have all been improved, perhaps as a direct result of the Patient's Charter (1992). Communication improvements for *all* are being attempted, identifiable by the striving for a more organised and improved quality of service provided in the clinical areas. This is visible in the introduction of systems of care delivery and clinical audit.

Nearly all of the areas reviewed were using recognised assessment tools to deliver care, for example, models of nursing linked with the nursing process and pressure assessment scales such as Waterlow.

More work is required in the areas of documentation, whether uni- or multidisciplinary, in the discharge planning of patients, and in the writing of care plans. The provision of care by and within wards/OPD needs to become more research based and focused. Staff's beliefs and attitudes indicate that the philosophy of care needs to be written to encompass their real beliefs and what they are trying to achieve and provide. Staff are not just making lists of objectives that are not realistic or achievable.

The named, qualified nurse needs further development in order to find more creative and appropriate methods of implementation and in order to be reflective about staff workload and activity.

Care planning needs to be revisited in individual wards/OPDs in order to find appropriate methods of assessing, delivering, and evaluating care. These should respond to the ever-increasing workload of staff and reduce the length of stay for patients. Reduction of written paperwork is essential in order to ensure that care plans are read and evaluated for all patients and not just regarded as a paper exercise.

In summary, the practice review has provided a foundation of strengths and weaknesses, which can be developed and expanded upon in the future. Nursing and midwifery in this organisation will need to continue to be creative and to reflect about the future in order to respond to the ever-increasing demands being made upon the high quality of service they already provide. This is to be facilitated through the implementation of the individual nursing development plans.

## STAGE 5: PROGRESS TO DATE

Individual nursing development plans have been drawn up, outlining areas requiring development in practice review. See, for example, Figure 3.12.

The sharing of ideas/experiences will be facilitated via the Practice Development Centre through the directorates' individual Practice Development Adviser. This will be in conjunction with the Ward/OPD Manager, Clinical Nurse Specialist, and their Director, who will work in collaboration with *all* staff to expand and enhance the standards and quality of care in their clinical areas. A smaller-scaled, stratified, random sample of clinical areas will be selected in which the practice review will be repeated. Its aim will be to measure the impact of education and training undertaken from the nursing development plans and its overall impact upon the clinical standards and quality in the organisation.

A summary of major findings was provided to all senior managers at the hospital's Professional Forum. Following the review, many areas of innovative practice have been implemented and documented in the

| N | Standard | Action required | Who | When | Start date | Date completed |
|---|----------|-----------------|-----|------|------------|----------------|
| 3 | Documentation | | | | | |

**Figure 3.12**

Nursing development plan

nursing press: McSherry (1996), Smith and Bassett (1996), Hepworth *et al.* (1996), McSherry *et al.* (1997), Haddock and Bassett (1996).

## THE VALUE OF THE PRACTICE REVIEW TO PRACTICE DEVELOPMENT

In light of the recent government White Papers (1997; 1998a, b) and the expressed need for all hospital and community trusts to establish a system of 'clinical governance'. the practice review supports the clinical governance agenda by providing:

- a framework that offers confidence to the public and staff in knowing that their local health services aim to offer quality standards of care that are both efficient and effective;
- assurance that standards and practices of care are based upon research evidence, in an attempt to minimise risks in the pursuit of clinical excellence and measurable patient outcomes.

The outlined practice review would be of little use in assisting hospital and community trusts to establish the existence of evidence-based care if used in isolation to record individual findings of directorates.

The practice review demonstrated the value of using a tailor-made measurement tool to evaluate the quality of care currently being delivered in the clinical area of nursing and midwifery. The results highlighted those issues requiring practice development and support in the future (key aspects of any clinical governance structures). A solid baseline indicator has been achieved for the quality departments to work from over the coming years. The practice review has met all the aims it set out to achieve. Where a baseline indicator of the trust's nursing and midwifery clinical practices was established against an agreed set of standards, many good/excellent practices have been highlighted and shared among the individual wards and directorates.

The framework of evaluating care delivery and organisational, education, corporate, professional, and care-planning systems proved to be an invaluable and workable template, which may be offered to other organisations to use to obtain an initial baseline indicator of standards and quality. Although the analysis and writing of this report has taken a great deal of time, the value and benefits will continue to be enjoyed in the future by the sustained implementation and evaluation of the individual nurse development plans.

## CONCLUSION

In conclusion it could be argued that practice development is everyone's business and is an integral part of an individual's professional accountability in the pursuit to improve standards through a process of lifelong learning and continued professional development. If you believe the latter to be true, advances or evaluations in practice must be dependent upon a mutual and respectful partnership between employees and employers to highlight the support needed and resources required to advance or evaluate a given aspect of an individual's or team's practice. The support could be in the form of individuals or teams with a remit to facilitate practice development, or linked to a department dedicated to quality management. Successful practice development depends upon the establishment of individual systems and processes to ensure that you can continue to develop professionally and you can measure and evaluate the effectiveness of your role in the organisation. There are a variety of ways and methods to help you achieve this goal. It is imperative that you utilise them. After all, practice development is about communication, collaboration, and the facilitation of individual, team, or organisational development through sharing and networking.

◀ **Key points**

- A strategy of how you intend to assess, implement, and evaluate the achievement of your key roles and responsibilities should be your number one priority.
- Practice development should be linked to continuous professional development, personal development plans, and the concept of lifelong learning.
- Practice development is everyone's business.
- Practice development requires systems and processes for proving individual, team, and organisational support.
- Structures and processes should be developed to measure and evaluate the impact of practice development upon an individual, team, or organisation.
- Practices are to be shared and disseminated.

**RECOMMENDED READING**

Bassett, C. (1999) *Clinical Supervision: A Guide for Implementation.* Nursing Times Books, London.
McGill, I. and Beaty, L. (1995) *Action Learning. A Guide for Professional, Management and Educational Development.* Kogan Page, London.
Page, S. (2001) Demystifying practice development. *Nursing Times* 97(22), 36–37.

**REFERENCES**

Bassett, C. (1995) The sky's the limit. *Nursing Standard* 9(39), 18–19.
Bassett, C. (1999) *Clinical Supervision: A Guide for Implementation.* Nursing Times Books, London.
Collins, W. (1987) *Collins Universal English Dictionary.* William Collins, Glasgow.
Cutcliffe, J. R. and Bassett, C. (1997) Introducing change in nursing: the case of research. *Journal of Nursing Management* 5, 241–247.
Department of Health (1993) *The Evolution of Clinical Audit.* DoH, London.
Department of Health (1997) *The New NHS: Modern and Dependable.* HMSO, London.
Department of Health (1998a) *A First Class Service: Quality in the New NHS.* HMSO, London.
Department of Health (1998b) *Achieving Effective Practice.* London.

Feely, M. (1999) *Benchmarking, Networking and Developing Best Practice.* Office for Health Management. http://.www.tohm.ie/news_may 99/maypg2.html

Haddock, J. and Bassett, C. (1996) Nurses' perception of reflective practice. *Nursing Standard* 11(32), 39–41.

Hepworth, S., Gaskill, T. and Bassett, C. (1996) An holistic approach to pain. *Nursing Standard* 10(17), 18–20.

Kohner, N. (1994) *Clinical Supervision: An Executive Summary.* King's Fund Centre, London.

Lathlean, J. (1999) *Directory of NDU Activities.* King's Fund Centre, London.

McGill, I. and Beaty, L. (1995) *Action Learning. A Guide for Professional, Management and Educational Development.* Kogan Page, London.

McSherry, R. (1996) Multidisciplinary approach to patient communication. *Nursing Times* 92(8), pp 42–43.

McSherry, R. and Haddock, J. (1999) Evidence based practice: its place within clinical governance. *British Journal of Nursing* 8(2), 114–117.

McSherry, R. and Pearce, P. (2002) *Clinical Governance. A Guide to Implementation for Healthcare Professionals.* Blackwell Scientific Publishers, Oxford.

McSherry, R., Bassett, C., Bond, M. and Mudge, K. (1997) A collaborative approach to research. *Nursing Times* 93(16), 50–51.

McSherry, R., Simmons, S. and Abbott, P. (2002) *Evidence-Informed Nursing: A Guide for Clinical Nurse.* Routledge, London.

National Health Service Executive (1999) Health Service Circular 1999/154 Continuing Professional Development: Quality in the NHS. DoH, London.

Page, S. (ed.) (1998) *The Practice Development Unit: An Experiment in Multi-disciplinary Innovation.* Whurr, London.

Page, S. (2001) Demystifying practice development. *Nursing Times* 97(22), 36–37.

Pearson, A., Wiles, A., Goldstone, L., Bradshaw, S. and Wainwright, P. (1987) *Nursing Quality Measurement: Quality Assurance Methods for Peer Review.* John Wiley, Chichester.

Sackett, L. D., Richardson, W. S., Rosenburg, W. and Haynes, B. R. (1997) *Evidence-Based Medicine: How to Practice & Teach EBM.* Churchill Livingstone, London.

Schroeder, P. S. and Maibusch, R. M. (1984) *Nursing Quality Assurance: A Unit Based Approach.* Aspen, Rochville, MD.

Smith, L. and Bassett, C. (1996) Parents in the post anaesthetic care unit. *Nursing Standard* 9(11), 32–34.

Wills, T. (2000) Practice development: restoring hope. *Elderly Care* 12(2), 29.

## USEFUL WEBSITES

Commission for Health Improvements:
www.chi.nhs.uk

European Quality Foundation Management:
www.forum2001.org

Investors in People:
www.iipuk.co.uk

# MANAGERIAL ISSUES IN PRACTICE DEVELOPMENT    4

*Carole Hopps*

## INTRODUCTION

Having read this book so far, I am sure you will agree that having a manager who is supportive of practice development and education, in ensuring continuous quality improvements of a service(s), founded upon the principles of evidence-based practiceis a very useful individual to have on your side. I have to admit I have been very fortunate in my career to have had supportive managers. If this is not the case in your area, fear not, for you can learn to manage your manager.

Why are the manager and managerial issues important? Because practice development needs managing. Practice development, like the individual, needs support, motivation, encouragement, power, and control. If you are not in a position to affect these elements, that is not a problem; it is just something you need to consider when thinking about practice development. Whatever skill you do not have or whichever resource is not available, it is sufficient to know someone who has that skill or resource. All of these issues are very important when you start to consider practice development. However, once you have changed something in practice, you will enjoy a sense of achievement. You will see yourself as a professional, along with your colleagues in the multidisciplinary team, putting theory into practice, making your practice evidence based, and affecting patient outcomes.

Practice development is important today and is incorporated into government initiatives such as clinical governance, audit, and clinical effectiveness and helps to provide that 'First Class Service' in the 'New NHS' of today (Department of Health [DoH], 1997; 1998).

So what is this chapter about? It is about making practice development and changes in practice happen and being realistic about the influence of the organisation and the individual. Change does not happen overnight. It is multifaceted and here we are going to consider some of the managerial issues that we may encounter along the way. This will be achieved using a problem-solving approach. Reflective questions will be posed and guidelines for practice will be provided. I would also recommend that you compile a portfolio of evidence as you work through this chapter. When I say 'portfolio' I do not mean typed up, always correctly spelt, and filed in a leather-bound case. I mean an A4 file for your personal use, where you will set down your thoughts, handwritten if you like. This documentation is for you and you may compile it however you wish. It could be in full form or note form. As long as you understand it, and can interact with it, that is what is important. This portfolio can then be used to compile your documentation of the process and can be used as a resource for future practice developments. It will also remind you of the work that you have produced and how much you have achieved. This is nothing additional to that which you are asked to do as a professional. But it will provide you with a useful point of reference. It may also be useful for Post-Registration Education and Practice (PREP) (NMC, 1990) or Continuing Professional Development (CPD) requirements.

The chapter will be structured by initially considering what skills you have and what skills you need to acquire. An area of practice will then be identified to work on while reading through the chapter. Afterwards this example will be used to explore the management of practice development and innovation. We will look at how the team can be motivated; what we need to make practice development happen; what style of management is required for the development; and how leadership styles can affect the development. We will then consider conflict, audit, professional development, and how we can measure what patient outcomes have been achieved through this practice development. To close the chapter a summary will be offered and implications for practice considered.

The key issues explored in this chapter are:

- managing change
- innovation
- management and leadership styles
- motivating the individual
- motivating the team
- including the multidisciplinary team
- conflict
- resources
- time management
- patient outcomes
- political influences
- audit
- professional development.

## Activity 4.1

Before you go any further it may be useful to consider what skills you already possess which will be of use to you while working through this chapter.

Pick up your portfolio and on one page write the skills that you possess and on a second page write the skills you need to develop or that you might wish to borrow from someone else. You may want to involve them in your project; if so, write their name by the side of the skill you think may be needed. If you experience any difficulties thinking of the skills, refer to the useful skills for managing practice development outlined in Box 4.1.

Now read on and compare your findings with the remaining sections of this chapter.

I can remember starting in one managerial post where I was expected to write many letters and reports. I had always considered myself not to be particularly good at writing and always found this particular task daunting. I therefore decided to enlist a senior colleague who worked in the department to help me whenever I had reports or letters to write. Her English was particularly good and I think she was surprised yet pleased that I felt able to ask and acknowledge that I needed help.

This is the way in which we as professionals can begin to foster collaboration in our practice with the multidisciplinary team. I hope this simple example from my own experience helps you realise that we may not all possess every skill we need to get a job done but we probably know someone who does.

Now you have identified the skill areas you want to develop and the skills of others you may wish to involve in the project, let's move onto an area to develop in practice.

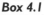
**Box 4.1**

---

Useful skills for managing practice development

- Communications skills
- Time management skills
- Power: individual, organisational, departmental
- Leadership skills
- Motivator
- Energy
- Know the team's characters and capabilities
- Enthusiasm
- Decision-making
- Problem solving
- Audit technique
- Evaluation

---

## THE DEVELOPMENT OF PRACTICE

Before we begin to look at the theories underpinning practice development and the issues arising from changing practice, I want you to think of an area in practice that you would like to change. If you cannot think of an element of practice, here are some suggestions and potential projects.

Think about the last time you were at work. During that time were there any problems that occurred or made you think about your practice? It might be a recurrent problem. Was there a question mark over something being done or not being done? It might be a practice issue, educational issue, research issue, or managerial issue. It might be something that incorporates all of these areas. Try to think of a patient scenario rather than something that affects the professional only. The reason I recommend this is that certain authors propose that we are too busy concentrating on our own development as professionals when it comes to practice development and we do not focus on the outcomes that can be achieved for the patient (Greenwood, 2000).

If you are having difficulty thinking of a practice issue, have a look at the statements from practice listed below. I have asked professionals from several specialities to identify practice issues. Here are some of the problems identified.

## STATEMENTS FROM PRACTICE FOR POTENTIAL DEVELOPMENT

*Nobody these days sees infection control as their problem. Ownership of the environment is the problem. I wonder what I could do to change this attitude?*

*The documentation used within this unit is complex and repetitive. What we need is single patient documentation.*

*I wonder if anyone else is interested in setting up an evidence-based practice group?*

*Patients should be allowed to administer their own medication.*

*Patients need more preparation for theatre. How can I introduce pre-operative visiting?*

*Communication and transfer of patients between wards is really problematic. I wonder if the rest of my colleagues feel this way?*

*Why do we not allow relatives or significant others to be present during resuscitation?*

*I have got a great idea for the retention and recruitment of staff.*

## PLANNING

Hopefully by now you will have identified an area of practice which you want to develop. If you have not, this is not a problem; you can still read this chapter of the book and examine the process of change and how a change in practice can be managed.

This particular phase of managing change is very important. It is, however, very time consuming and can be frustrating. What do I need? Who will help? Is anyone else interested? These are all questions I have asked myself on many an occasion. At this stage what I often find it useful to use is Rudyard Kipling's (1993) six honest serving men. These are: Who? What? Where? When? Why? and How?

You can refer back to your portfolio and write these headings down. Then you can start to consider and plan your change. You may want to start with What? What do I want to change? Then you may ask yourself: Why do I want to change that practice? At this stage, if you are working on your own still, you may find it useful to find some evidence that supports what you believe the problem to be. You may even ask the advice of others. What do they think? However, do not be put off at this stage if some people disagree with you. This is quite common and we will consider this when discussing change. You will also get some people saying things like 'If it is not broken, why fix it?' and in some instances they may be right. Others may say, 'There is no point in trying to change X. Many people have tried and it has not worked.' Maybe it was not that the practice did not need changing but the way the change was approached.

You can then continue with the six honest serving men. Where is the change going to happen? Who will help me with the change? When will I implement the process? The timescale may be movable unless of course something has to be changed by a given date. The main thing is to consider all of these points and take your time getting to a position where you can commence the change in practice. I have not forgotten the How? Hopefully the rest of this chapter will examine how, identifying what else you need to consider, and will assist you in making that change happen. Remember to be patient: change does not happen overnight. Also, choose a small project; it is amazing how the project will grow.

**Box 4.2**

> You could also use a process to plan change that all nurses are familiar with:
>
> - Assess
> - Plan
> - Implement
> - Evaluate
>
> Lowe (1995) adopts a similar approach using a diagnostic assessment:
>
> - Identify
> - Diagnose
> - Assess
>
> Use whichever approach works best for you and your area of practice

## MOTIVATING THE MULTIDISCIPLINARY TEAM

When motivating the multidisciplinary team, according to Hunt (1992), you need to consider three things:

- the goal
- the energy
- the reward.

Different things motivate different people. The goal of the individual needs to be known. If the goal is not shared then this may not allow the change in practice to be achieved. Also, where do the individuals concerned use their energy? Is their energy directed towards this change in practice or do they have another agenda (Jolley and Brykczynska, 1993)? Last and by no means least, we all need a reward after hard work. Rewards differ from person to person. They do not have to be money orientated. The reward might be about achievement of the goal or it might be seeing the change in practice implemented or recognition of the achievement by others. However, an individual's preferred reward may be money and you need to consider whether this project will achieve any reward for that individual. If not, it might be better not to include them in the development. Hopefully, for professionals some reward will come from knowing that practice has been changed for the better and has had a positive effect on patient outcome.

When considering motivation, Herzberg (1974) categorises individuals' jobs as satisfiers/motivators and dissatisfiers/hygiene factors (Box 4.3). Herzberg explains that the hygiene factors can be satisfied or met as needs for individuals but at no point do they become motivators and only the motivators listed can motivate. Therefore you may find it useful when trying to motivate people to emphasise the motivators identified by Herzberg.

**Box 4.3**

---

Motivational influences (Herzberg, 1974)

*Motivators/satisfiers*
- Achievement
- Recognition
- Work itself
- Responsibility
- Role Advancement

*Hygiene/dissatisfiers*
- Company policy and administration
- Supervision
- Salary
- Interpersonal relations at work
- Working conditions

---

Getting people involved and motivated initially can be time consuming and frustrating. However, when you do get people on your side and you do realise that other people have the same interests or want to get involved this, in turn, moves you one step forward. It is also useful to know at this stage who is not interested, since these people may need consideration when the practice development is introduced. This will be considered in more depth when we look at change and innovation.

It is exceptionally important to know the individuals that you work with. As identified earlier in this chapter, one of the key skills for practice development is knowing the capabilities and characters of the team. You may actively seek out like-minded people who you know are rewarded by practice development and who are interested in the area that you wish to consider.

Take a few minutes now to refer to your portfolio. Consider your practice development. Are you sure what your goal is? Where do you get your energy? What will be your reward? It may be useful to consider these points. You may also at this stage wish to think about who you need to get involved from inside and outside the department. Do not exclude people at this point who you think may not want this change to happen. All the more reason to include them.

> *I can remember once in practice being involved in a practice development. I was an inexperienced manager of change and to my folly I did not involve a group of people who this change in practice specifically effected. They did not get involved in the change because I excluded them. They waited until the change was introduced and then placed several barriers in the way. Needless to say, the change did not happen. What is more, it was now twice as difficult to introduce the change, as the group that had been excluded now did not want to be involved.*

Remember to make sure your team is multidisciplinary. At this stage it is also useful to approach other people and ask their opinion and to start to look for people who are influential. Start to canvas for your campaign.

Depending on your position in the organisation you may also find it useful at this stage to inform your line manager about what you are considering. Can they help? Will they actively not help? Do they know anyone else who has already looked at this development? As the saying goes, do not try to reinvent the wheel.

I am also aware that some trusts today keep databases of individuals who are specifically interested in certain areas of practice. Does your department/organisation have such a database? Be prepared to share ideas.

Now we have had a few thoughts about the practice development and started to plan the change, we must take time to consider the management of change.

## MANAGING CHANGE, INNOVATION, AND THE CHANGE AGENT

As previously stated, change needs managing. It can be managed in many different ways, so it would seem reasonable first to consider change strategy and theory, since several approaches are available. When it comes to models of change, very little has changed. In this section of the chapter you will find some old favourites. When I have thought it appropriate, I have introduced some newer models. However, as Menix *et al.* (2000) point out, the newer ones are about strategic management and political influences, in contrast to the older linear models that are often used.

At the start of this chapter we considered the skills required to manage practice development, what it was we wanted to change about practice, and the process of planning. This section of the chapter is about implementing the change. The next section therefore will cover managing change, management styles, conflict, time management, and resource requirements.

As stated, several options for change strategy are available. One commonly cited is that described by Bennis *et al.* (1976). These authors describe three approaches to change: rational-empirical, power coercive, and normative re-educative. Do not be put of by the terminology. The three approaches are simply defined in Box 4.4.

**Box 4.4**

---

Change theories (Bennis *et al.*, 1976)

*Rational-empirical*
This change strategy is top-down in its approach. It works on the premise that if sufficient evidence is available about the need to change practice, then the individual will want to change.

*Power coercive*
Again a top-down approach, which assumes that knowledge is power and that position is power and that individuals can use these skills to influence individuals who do not have as much power.

*Normative re-educative*
This strategy is a bottom-up approach. Individuals identify in their working practice the need for change, much as you are doing by reading this book.

---

Having considered these approaches to change management, you may wish to look back at your identified practice development and decide which approach may best suit you. You may wish, using your portfolio, to identify some changes that have taken place in your department, unit, or ward and decide which approach was used. Some examples are: the identification of hazard safety bulletins, day-to-day interaction with a superior, and shared governance.

I would argue that the normative re-educative approach is the best approach for practice development. I think it sits nicely with continued professional development, evidence-based practice, clinical effectiveness, autonomous practice, and clinical governance. This approach is described by Burnes (1996) as an emergent approach to change and acknowledges that change does not have to be management led.

Rather than make a list of all of the change strategies and models that are available I decided to refer to current articles that have been published in the multidisciplinary health care arena to identify models and strategies that have been used in practice. I hope that from among these published examples from practice you will be able to choose an approach that is useful to you. Also these articles prove that change can work.

A much quoted author on the management of change is Lewin (1958). Lewin identifies three stages in the change process: unfreezing, moving, and refreezing. The process does not necessarily move from one stage to another in a straightforward fashion. Sometimes there is movement back and forth or the change process can get stuck at one stage. Neal (1995) uses this approach in an article about change in practice. Lewin's force field analysis is also used to consider the driving and restraining forces in relation to the change and may help further identify things that will help and things that will hinder.

A personal favourite of mine is a diagnostic model of change presented by Nadler and Tushman (1977). This diagnostic model is presented in a diagrammatic form and considers that the department/ area of practice has an internal environment but also has an environment outside the clinical area. The environment outside the department is divided into social, economical, and political facets. As health care professionals, we do not always consider the external influences and how they affect our professional working lives.

The internal environment of the practice area has four parts: the task, the individuals, the formal organisational arrangements, and the informal culture. Additionally, Nadler and Tushman acknowledge that leadership is important in any change process and that the parts of the internal environment must share the vision of change with the leader and vice versa.

Barnes (1995) uses the Nadler and Tushman model in a case study. This article is referenced so that you can consider an example from practice and observe the model's practical application and its use in analysis of a situation. Alternatively, you may wish to analyse your own change.

The model also includes the culture of the individuals working in the clinical area. I consider this to be important and yet not many models of change consider it. Culture is important and can affect or even halt changes in practice. A study of particular interest here is one that was completed on behalf of the English National Board (ENB, 1996). This research studied newly qualified nurses who had completed Project 2000 training and asked about applying theory to practice. The nurses in the sample felt they wanted to fit in to the ward rather than change practice, because they had a need to belong.

This is a prime example of how culture can effect changes in practice. From experience I would say this is an area that is often overlooked. Please do not be put off by this example. Often when change is being considered it is important to identify the potential stumbling blocks. Remember the old adage: forewarned is forearmed. Another approach to managing change could be a SWOT analysis. 'SWOT' is an acronym for 'strengths, weaknesses, opportunities, threats'. Write on a piece of paper these four headings at the top of four columns. Then, referring to your portfolio, write down under each heading any strengths, opportunities, weaknesses, and threats that pertain to your chosen practice development. This model can be used to clarify thoughts, identify individuals committed to the project, and compare the positive elements of the development and the areas for improvement. Bailey and Cassidy (1996) use a SWOT analysis approach when considering a change in practice. You may once again find this useful to obtain and examine how they used it in practical application.

A newer model is one developed by Carney (2000). This model was developed through the use of a focus group. The model has five building blocks: critical success factors for change, communication process, acceptance or resistance to change, implementation process, and evaluation process. Each building block has seven key variables, which are sentences that direct the individual managing or evaluating the change. The change management model also has a measurement constructs tool, which can be used in conjunction with the model to score each variable. The measurement constructs tool was adapted from a tool described by Clarke and Garside (1997). I think it is comprehensive, easy to follow, and is specific to health care practice. An added bonus is that the tool can be used for evaluation and scores can be attributed to each key variable.

This model hopefully provides you with an updated version from practice and demonstrates that older models can be adapted and used in practice today. If you find a model that you like but you feel there are elements missing, then add them. Make the model useful in practice and specific for your needs. Many different approaches can be used to manage change. You may find that you want to use several models or devise your own from the examples given. Whatever you decide, choose an approach that suits you and the area you practice in.

## Innovation

Rogers (1962) identified that individuals respond in different ways to innovation and change. Rogers' diagrammatic representation of this response categorises individuals as: 2% innovators, 13% early adopters, 34% early majority, 35% late majority, and 16% laggards. The innovators are people who might bring about change. Early adopters are people who readily accept change. The early majority accept change but not necessarily that readily. The late majority are the sceptics and the laggards will not accept change and may even try to sabotage it and stop it happening. There are also those who may vote with their feet and leave because they are not at ease with the change.

I have found this kind of information useful in my management career: the knowledge that a change even if managed correctly is not going to please everybody.

Take a moment and consider a change in practice that has been introduced recently. Using Rogers' categories as guidelines, which category did you fit in, in relation to the change? Having been involved in a lot of changes in practice, I know that at different times I have fitted in every category.

Only the other day I was using Rogers' model to help a student to analyse a change that had happened in practice. She found it interesting that when she had tried to introduce a change, one person she thought would be for the change was actually against it. This is not an uncommon experience when you are introducing change. It can be overcome by quickly getting the individual involved with the change or, even better, by asking who would like to be involved before the change is introduced.

## Change agents

A change agent is defined as an expert who manages change (Wright, 1994). I am unsure about the word 'expert'. I think the change agent could also be someone who aspires to be an expert. Perhaps an individual like yourself who is reading this book to gain skills that will help with practice development and will maybe become an expert.

A change agent needs to be familiar with all aforementioned theories and processes. A change agent needs to know the people, the organisation, and who to involve outside the organisation, for example in higher education, so that they can bring people in as and when they are needed. A change agent also needs to be aware of management and leadership styles.

## MANAGEMENT AND LEADERSHIP STYLES

What is your style of management? What is the management style of your manager? Refer to your portfolio and write them down. If you are not familiar with management terminology, then write down the characteristics of your style of management. Try then to say what is good and bad about the styles. Are they very different? Are they very similar?

Now you have completed this exercise, let's look at some styles of management and leadership which have been defined. Lewin (1958) defined leadership styles as autocratic where the manager decides, democratic where decisions are made after discussion, and *laissez-faire* where there is a group approach to management. Hersey and Blanchard (1982) describe the manager's actions as a means of management style and divide them into four categories: telling, selling, delegating, and participating. I think there are definite similarities here with the leadership styles defined by Lewin (see Figure 4.1). Which styles do you think equate to the categories of Hersey and Blanchard?

Do any of these definitions describe what you have written in your portfolio? I have worked with all of the types of managers described. When I was less experienced as a manager I had one management style and stuck to it. Years later I remember being irritated with myself when I realised that I could use different approaches for different situations. Why had I not done this before? I then realised that I had not done this before because earlier in my career I did not have the skills to move between different styles.

This example will hopefully convince you that there are different management styles that can be adopted but overall you will feel more comfortable with one style over another. Adopt that style and move in

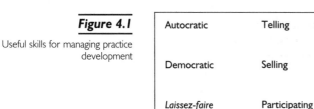

**Figure 4.1**

Useful skills for managing practice development

| | |
|---|---|
| Autocratic | Telling |
| Democratic | Selling |
| *Laissez-faire* | Participating |
| | Delegating |

and out of other styles if you can but only if you feel happy doing so. Remember, stick to what you know.

Further, in clinical practice today, and certainly for managing change, I would suggest that individuals prefer a manager who will discuss issues with them and will involve them in decision-making processes. At times there are changes that need to be declared rather than discussed, such as safety bulletins or information about a product that is to be withdrawn.

## CONFLICT

When you introduce or try to manage a change in practice there is a good chance, as discussed, that some people will not like the change. This can cause conflict between individuals or groups and between the introducer of the change (you) and individuals involved in the change.

Although conflict is a fact of life, it can be managed and resolved (Banner, 1995). One thing to remember is, wherever possible, do not ignore conflict, since it will not be ignored (DiPaola and Hoy, 2001). Conflict can be difficult to address but it can equally be difficult to identify. Conflict can be destructive but it can also be positive and beneficial to practice (Banner, 1995). Some authors would argue that it is required to aid innovation and change (DiPaola and Hoy, 2001).

Hopefully, this section will give you some methods to identify conflict and go some way to enabling you to deal with conflict. I can remember being a less experienced manager when I first became a Sister. An incident occurred in practice that required me to speak to a member of staff about their behaviour. I thought about my approach long and hard and it caused me some anxiety. In the end, having let the time between incident and talk lapse a little too long, I had a chat with the member of staff concerned. The meeting went better than I had expected and the staff member was pleased that I had talked to them rather than ignoring it because they too felt they had handled the incident badly. I was so relieved about the positive outcome of this meeting. However, I now know it could have been so different, depending on the staff member's response. Now when I identify a conflict situation it causes me more anguish to leave it alone than it does to deal with the situation. Conflict does not go away, it does not get better for being left, and it is better dealt with, for the sooner you identify it the sooner it can be resolved or managed.

So, how can you identify conflict? According to Handy (1985) the causes of conflict are: poor communication, inter-group hostility and jealousy, inter-group friction, escalation of arbitration, proliferation of rules and regulations, and low morale. Therefore if you identify any of these happening when you are introducing a change, then you need to be aware that there is some conflict that requires resolving or managing.

Thomas (1976) describes avoidance, competition, collaboration, accommodation, and compromise as five ways of handling conflict. Avoidance is ignoring the conflict. Competition is wanting to win. The other three – accommodation, compromise, and collaboration – involve working together and working through the conflict to a positive end.

Heaney (2001) suggests a simple yet straightforward approach to resolving conflict. He suggests that the individual managing the conflict should think positively, be open, explain the situation, separate the personal from the professional, avoid anger, and put things behind you after the event. This is good common sense; it is so easy to make situations more difficult when dealing with conflict. Heaney's framework is simple and reminds the individual of the skills required to calm down a situation. This approach may also be of use to you in practice, since change is not the only thing that causes conflict.

## TIME MANAGEMENT AND RESOURCES

Timescales are very important. Management of your own and others' time is particularly necessary. How many times do you hear people say 'if I only had the time'? I do live in the real world and I do realise that time is precious in practice. Which is all the more reason why time has to be managed well. Make sure you identify how long things will take and be realistic. Identify what is needed. Go back to the start of the chapter and use Mr Kipling's 'six honest serving men' again. From these you can make a plan and get together the individuals you need to help you make the chosen change happen. Out of courtesy you should let your manager know what is happening. You may find that they will provide you with some resources. Most of all, be enthusiastic: it is contagious.

## EVALUATION AND AUDIT

An essential ingredient that health care professionals, teams, and organisations often neglect to include when developing or reviewing new or existing ways of working is evaluation. The Collins dictionary defines 'evaluate' as 'to find the value or amount of; to judge the quality of; appraise'. To demonstrate the value of practice development in health and social care settings, the inclusion of ways to evaluate the impact a new innovation or service development has had on individual, team, or organisational performance is crucial. In practice development, performance can be measured and evaluated in a variety of ways: audits, user satisfaction surveys, comparative benchmarking, to name but a few.

Evaluation in this instance is about highlighting or reducing clinical risks, and promoting continuous quality improvement. The challenge facing many health care professionals, teams, or organisations with a remit to promote or advance practice is to choose the best method to evaluate the efficiency and effectiveness of a change in practice. Chapter 3 outlined a variety of ways to make this process easier.

### PROFESSIONAL DEVELOPMENT: WHAT HAVE YOU LEARNT?

Take a moment to consider how you have developed professionally and what you have learnt. Write this down in your portfolio once you have implemented and evaluated the change in question. You might be surprised by some of the things you have learnt. There will be some you expected and others that were definite bonuses.

Some learning experiences may have been difficult or challenging but you will definitely have learnt something. Remember to record this for PREP requirements. Perhaps you could also think about informing others or try to get your practice development published.

If you experience difficulties in writing down what you have learnt, just put a heading 'I have learnt' and then list the areas you feel have developed.

### PATIENT OUTCOMES

Consider how your practice development has influenced patient outcomes. If your practice development was more about your development than affecting patient outcomes then perhaps you could consider how the skills you have learnt could affect patient outcomes. Write these thoughts down in your portfolio.

### CONCLUSION

In this chapter we have considered the management of change, innovation, management and leadership styles, and motivating the individual and the multidisciplinary team. Here are some implications for practice and some key points to remember and consider.

### Implications for practice

If change can be introduced into practice and managed effectively, our practice will become more evidence based. All wards and units could become practice development units. Patient outcomes could be improved through evidence-based practice. Care could really become team orientated. Professional practice could move forward. Individuals, teams, and organisations will learn to live with change and become more familiar with change management.

- Involve the team.
- Know the individuals you work with and how change affects people.
- Know your management style.
- Think of what skills you possess to manage change.
- Borrow skills from other people if you do not have them.
- Resources and time management are as important as people.
- Keep motivated.
- Conflict identification and management.

---

Broome, A. (1998) *Managing Change*, 2nd edn. Macmillan, Basingstoke.

**RECOMMENDED READING**

---

Bailey, J. and Cassidy, A. (1996) Using theory to introduce change in practice. *Nursing Times* 10(51), 40–43.

Banner, D. K. (1995) Conflict resolution: a recontextualization. *Leadership and Organizational Development Journal* 16(1), 31–34.

Barnes, P. C. (1995) Management for doctors. Managing Change *British Medical Journal* 310, 6979, 590–592.

Bennis, W. G., Benne, K. D., Chin, R. and Corey, K. E. (1976) *The Planning of Change*. Holt, Rinehart & Winston, London.

Broome, A. (1998) *Managing Change*, 2nd edn. Macmillan, Basingstoke.

Burnes, B. (1996) No such thing as a 'one best way' to manage organizational change. *Management Decision* 34(10), 11–18.

Carney, M. (2000) The development of a model to manage change; reflection on a critical incident in a focus group setting. An innovative approach. *Journal of Nursing Management* 8(5), 265–272.

Clarke, A. and Garside, J. (1997) The development of a best practice model of change management. *European Management Journal* 15(5), 537–545.

Department of Health (1997) *The New NHS: Modern, Dependable*. HMSO, London.

Department of Health (1998) *A First Class Service: Quality in the New NHS*. HMSO, London.

DiPaola, M. F. and Hoy, W. K. (2001) Formalization, conflict and change: constructive and destructive consequences in schools. *International Journal of Educational Management* 15(5), 238–244.

English National Board (1996) *Research Highlights. Project 2000: Perceptions of the Philosophy and Practice of Nursing*. No. 17. ENB, London.

Greenwood, J. (2000) Clinical development units (nursing): issues surrounding their establishment and survival. *International Journal of Nursing Practice* 6(6), 338–344.

Handy, C. B. (1985) *Understanding Organizations*. Penguin, London.

Heaney, L. F. (2001) A question of management: conflict, pressure and time. *International Journal of Educational Management* 15(4), 197–203.

Hersey, P. and Blanchard, K. (1982) *Management of Organization Behaviour*, 4th edn. Prentice Hall, Hemel Hempstead.

Herzberg, F. (1974) *Work and the Nature of Man*. Crosby Lockwood Staples, London.

Hunt, J. W. (1992) *Managing People at Work. A Manager's Guide to Behaviour in Organisations*. McGraw Hill, London.

**REFERENCES**

Jolley, M. and Brykczynska, G. (1993) *Nursing It Hidden Agendas*. Edward Arnold, London.

Kendrick, K., Weir, P. and Rosser, E. (1995) *Innovations in Nursing Practice*. Edward Arnold, London.

Kipling, R. (1993) *Just so Stories*. Wordsworth, Ware, UK.

Lewin, K. (1958) The group decisions and social change. In E. Maccoby (ed.), *Readings in Social Psychology*. Holt, Rinehart & Whinston, London. Cited in Kendrick, 1995.

Lowe, R. (1995) How to think change. *Nursing Management* 1(10), 12–13

Nadler, D. and Tushman, M. L. (1977) *Perspectives of Behaviour*. McGraw Hill, New York. Cited in Barnes, 1995.

Neal, K. (1995) Managing change: the named nurse. *Nursing Standard* 9(23), 29–30.

Rogers, E. M. (1962) *Diffusion of Innovations*. Free Press, New York. Cited in Wright 1994.

Thomas, K. W. (1976) Conflict and Conflict Management. In M. D. Dunnette (ed.), *Handbook of Industrial and Organizational Psychology*. Rand McNally, Chicago.

United Kingdom Central Council for Nursing, Midwifery and Health Visiting (1990) *Report of the Post-Registration Education and Practice Project*. London.

Wright, S. G. (1994) *Changing Nursing Practice*. Edward Arnold, London.

USEFUL WEBSITES

www.show.scot.nhs.uk/sign/
www.leeds.ac.uk/healthcare
www/mailbase.ac.uk/lists/practice-development-alliance

# Exploring the Barriers to Practice Development

# 5

*Bernie Wallis and Tina Long*

## Introduction

Initiating and sustaining practice development is fraught with obstacles, presenting the practitioner with challenges that may at times seem insurmountable. Being able to recognise and understand the nature and form of the barriers that may occur in developing practice is necessary in order to overcome them and achieve change. The first part of this chapter considers the appropriateness of change models as a framework for continuous improvement in practice. The problems of introducing developments in practice are explored and barriers identified and whole systems, culture, leadership, teamwork, and the involvement of patients and users are considered. A number of questions are then posed for you to consider and activities are presented to help explore the barriers identified in your own area of work.

## The problems of introducing practice development

A number of barriers and problems exist when one is introducing practice change. We have grouped these into five key areas: change models, culture, leadership, teams/team-working, and the patient/user perspective.

## The relevance of change models

Many traditional change models do not lend themselves to the continuous improvement essential in today's world. Models such as Lewin's (1951) were developed when the environment in which we worked was more predictable and stable. These approaches served us well for many years, but in the current climate of inter-agency working and working across professional and organisational boundaries a whole new mindset is required. The traditional approach has been to break organisations and teams down to their constituent parts rather than viewing them as a whole. An approach that has been around for some years but has gained momentum as a meaningful way of leading change is the whole systems approach. Pratt *et al.* (1999) uses the following definition: 'whole system working helps people make organisational connections that enable them to find sustainable solutions to local concerns. These connections are both with people and ideas.'

Often the issues that face health professionals are complex and require the abilities of more than one person if real solutions are to be found. In the past we have relied upon better planning, more efficient organising, controlling, and problem solving, all of which produce a degree of change and predictability. Although these elements still have an important part to play in any organisation, Kotter (1990) argues that these are all management functions, whereas to produce dramatic change one needs to establish direction, align people, motivate, and inspire, which are functions of leadership. Perhaps the mistake we have made in the past is to try to manage change, hence models of change management, rather than leading change.

Developing practice is about innovation and organisational learning. The evidence suggests that organisations are not good at learning and sustaining innovation. Schein (1996) argues that all organisations have a number of subcultures, which are not aligned to each other, and this lack of alignment hinders organisational learning. He goes on to highlight that these occupational cultures often do not understand each other and work at cross-purposes. This certainly has been the case in health care, different professional groups rarely getting together to understand each other's roles and values and to find some common ground. Only when we start to see the whole and not just our own view of the world do we begin to recognise the complexity and diversity of care provision.

Many of the change models of the past have been based on a mechanistic view that understanding the parts leads to an under-standing of the whole and that there is a linear relationship between the parts which is often hierarchical. Mintzberg and Jorgensen (1987) argue that the dominance of this sort of model hinders organisations' capacity to adapt and learn. In the past we have often implemented fixes for problems encountered in our day-to-day practice rather than seeking new ways of developing which recognise the complexity of many issues. We do not work in simple organisations; often we work in systems that are a mess, and we frequently try to simplify things to make them manageable. Stacey (1996) describes this organisational mess as important to success. He argues that 'the tension between stability and instability (challenging the status quo) leads to success'. According to this view we should be challenging the *status quo* and looking for new ways around problems.

One approach to new ways around problems is to view the organisation as a living system: a living system is made of a web of relationships and communication. The organisation is seen as being alive and value is placed on relationships both formal and informal. The richness of these connections will unleash ideas and innovation in the team. Effective development of practice can therefore only occur if this approach is adopted at the heart of the organisation. The practitioner therefore needs to consider change models that encompass this notion of whole living systems. The principles of this type of approach are essential to capture the complex relationships and interdependence of the many facets of developing practice.

## ORGANISATIONAL CULTURE

Culture is a complex matter, not always easy to understand, but it is a vital ingredient of any organisation. It is difficult to give one definition but many authors define culture as something that emerges from values and beliefs (Schein, 1996). It can therefore be defined as the assumptions, values, and beliefs that underpin an organisation and therefore determine the way that it behaves. These often lie beneath the surface and are sometimes difficult to determine, but are shared by members of the organisation and accepted by newcomers as the way things are.

The literature is ambiguous about the factors that cause culture to form. Research carried out by Hofstede (1990) provides evidence that staff perceptions of daily practices determine the core of an organisation's culture. If the notion of developing practice is central to the organisation and something in which everyone believes, one can begin to see how a culture of developing practice might emerge. On the other hand if this is not valued, then it becomes very difficult for one individual to try to develop practice.

In order for practice development to be effective there has to be a culture of empowerment. This means changing the way in which power and control are used in an organisation. Wallach (1993) suggests that cultures can be placed in three categories:

- bureaucratic
- innovative
- supportive.

Bureaucratic cultures do not facilitate the notion of practice development, whereas innovative and supportive cultures do. A crucial element, therefore, of developing a culture that will facilitate practice development is to determine the type of culture required and set out a strategy to develop such a culture. In organisations we pay a great deal of attention to the structure and the systems we put in place and yet often ignore the crucial element of developing the culture.

The sharing of values, beliefs, and attitudes is necessary for culture to be formed. The culture of an organisation is closely aligned to its strategy. If we really want to achieve our goal of developing practice, then we must align the strategy to do this with the culture required to make it possible. It may be that more than one culture exists in an organisation or a team. Subcultures often emerge, particularly where a number of different professional groups work together. Rituals, symbols, and myths often reinforce a particular culture. If change is enforced without dealing with these unconscious elements of the organisation, the underlying culture will eventually emerge.

## LEADERSHIP

Bass and Avolio (1993) highlight the relationship between organisational culture and leadership. Effective leaders change culture by understanding it first, then fostering a culture of creative change based on a new vision, values, and beliefs through facilitation and developing everyone to their full potential. One of the key barriers therefore in developing practice is a lack of strong leadership that uses an approach suited to working with uncertainty and complexity. Kotter (1990) differentiates between two broad types of leadership. Firstly, transactional leadership or management creates order and consistency and is concerned with coping with complexity, whereas Bass's model of transformational leadership is concerned with establishing direction, motivating and inspiring others, coping, and often producing major changes that are necessary to survive in new environments. Kotter's distinction reveals the leader/manager concerned with delegation, control, and retention of power. Transformational leadership in comparison is collaborative and consultative, places trust in the team members, and empowers them, as power is distributed evenly in relation to staff knowledge and experience. Although there is some form of control in transformational leadership, all members of the team are made to feel valued contributors. Hence transformational leadership appears to be more consistent with the prerequisites for developing practice.

Strong leadership can help the team develop shared visions and lead team members into becoming proactive and take responsibility for change. Having a shared vision, according to Goddard and Lenhardt (2000), allows control of complex systems and lends meaning to the development and the problems or failures that can occur at each stage of change. These authors go on to associate transformational leadership with co-responsibility, describing this dynamic of co-responsibility or shared governance based on a vision shared with team members as 'collective intelligence'. The logic of collective intelligence, they argue, enables an organisation to focus on the client's or patient's needs. The need for the organisation and leader to maximise the capacity for intelligent action, encouraging the use of intelligence and initiative by staff, can make the organisation more effective. Cowley (1999, 15) associates this with 'the ability to challenge values, norms, policies and underlying assumptions that may cause difficulties rather than aim to solve problems that present themselves'. They highlight the importance of having a deep understanding of the ethical basis of practical action. As practice development always involves a degree of risk taking, strong leadership requires a clear sense of ethical decision-making associated with such risks. Effective leaders also use intuition to inform their decision-making. When considered within the context of making clinical judgements intuition is associated with critical skills (Polge, 1995), whilst Miller (1995) associates such intuitive practice with risk taking.

A lack of appropriate leadership skills may become apparent both at the outset of the development and when the development reaches certain critical points or encounters obstacles if there is an inability to 'think outside of the box' and encourage this in others. The 'box' according to Dubrin (2001) confines and restricts thinking. The ability to think outside of the box may involve further risk taking, since it is often associated with creative and innovative thinking in the team. Problems will be encountered if the leadership does not facilitate such development among team members, which also involves ensuring the team has creative thinkers and utilises the ensuing outputs effectively. A further problem that may be encountered is a lack of professional development in the practice environment and/or the notion that practice development is not an integral part of the professional development of the team members. A lack of appropriate professional development to enable staff to initiate or engage in a change innovation may well be readily recognised by staff themselves. Strong leadership also requires facilitation, negotiation, critical reflection, and evaluation skills to ensure the success of the development and provide a coordinated and systematic approach as highlighted by McCormack (1999).

Identifying, developing, and supporting the needs of leaders in the organisation is vital as they search for and create opportunities to develop practice. A fundamental barrier, however, may be a lack of appropriate support from the top of the organisation both for those leading a development and for the development itself. This may hinder motivation and commitment in developing and sustaining change and in addressing resources issues. Practical resource problems can emerge, such as the time required, ensuring the leader is free to facilitate, having the appropriate expertise in the team, funding, or ready access to information sources. Although a lack of any of these resources can be a genuine barrier in some cases, resource problems are frequently used as an excuse for not developing practice. Support from the top of the organisation can create or remove potential barriers related to the scale of the change, since it can be too ambitious and the leader can become overawed by the scale of the change required or expected. Cowley (1999, 15) acknowledges 'the sheer complexity and inter-relatedness of the systems in which [we] work can seem so daunting that achieving small changes within known parameters can overwhelm'. The scale of the change will have a direct impact on resources, including the size of team involved in making the change and the associated challenges in nurturing and developing the team and changing the culture.

Finally, a lack of understanding of how the politics in the organisation impacts on practice development may also be a weakness of the leadership. An inability or lack of skills to engage with the politics and associated processes of networking and influencing others will be a potential barrier to the development. It is vital to understand the competing agendas and power dynamics of the organisation and where the power bases lie, particularly if a multi-professional team is central to the development. According to Wedwenburn Tate (1999), power and leadership in an inter-professional team should be shared between members depending on needs. The agenda of the new NHS (National Health Service) is clearly set within a far more multidisciplinary, multi-agency, and cooperative organisational framework than ever before.

Consequently, as Edwards and Hale (1999, 180) state, 'there is no automatic right to leadership in any sphere whatever the aspirations of the professions'. But what of the needs and power of patients and carers in practice change?

## INVOLVING PATIENTS AND USERS

All too often professionals think they know best and do not really engage patients and users in helping to develop practice. We all work within our own framework of meaning and assume that others, whether other professionals or patients, understand our viewpoint. Deigling *et al.* (1998) point to the fact that 'in naming and framing the world in medical-clinical terms medical clinicians ... create information about a reality which is in keeping with their perspective of what is central to the provision of care'. They go on to highlight that patients lack access to the information sets generated by other groups and are hence not in a position to counter the realities that these constitute. Patients are also not in a position to give perspectives on what they regard as important to the provision of care. Engaging these key people in practice development initiatives gives them a real opportunity to help shape services from their perspective and to enable them to be empowered as active participants in this process.

The relationships that often exist between professionals and patients are not empowering but actually disempowering. Deigling *et al.* (1998) describe this as patients being 'disenfranchised by the structures of power which characterise relations in the clinical setting'. The example used relates to patient records and describes the record as something central to care but a document that is always written from the perspective of the clinician, whether that be the nurse or the doctor. Very often patients are an absent voice in their own record of care. There are instances where this is no longer the case, but these are still few and far between. One way of engaging patients and users in the development of care is to utilise a process review approach to re-engineer the pathway of care. There are examples where this has proved to be very successful in enabling patients to help to identify short-comings in health care systems and to design innovative ways of delivering care. One such example is South Tees Hospitals NHS Trust, where a process review approach is taken when reshaping services. A whole systems event is held at which staff of all professional groups and grades sit around the table with patients and users of the service to map the patient journey through the system, identify real and potential failures in the current system, and finally redesign and implement the changes. Pratt *et al.* (1999) emphasise the point that 'people from different organisational cultures or professions find it hard to hear and respect the values of another group and reaching agreement on common ground is not an easy task'. If one adds the additional dimension of patients and users of the service, then the importance of getting people to share experiences and views cannot be under-estimated.

# Teams and Team-Working

An initial stage in initiating any practice change is to be clear who the team comprises, whether the innovation is being implemented by one individual or at a team level. There should be a clearly defined role in the team for patient and carer involvement. Gorman (1998) challenges teams about their ability to respond flexibly to different patient demands.

The context of patient care and therefore of practice initiatives is multidisciplinary whether the change is focused on one or several disciplines. Professional ideologies and cultures are often a barrier to successful change and can discourage change initiatives that require the active involvement of a multidisciplinary team. This often restricts innovation to being discipline specific, potentially limiting the impact on patient care. There are, according to Gorman (1998, 2), 'too many multi-disciplinary workplaces that are dominated by organisational and professional jealousies and conflict and they are undermined by a weak understanding of the processes at work beneath the surface'. There is a need therefore to understand the range, mix, and inherent problems within teams. In particular, multidisciplinary teams as professional preoccupations and inter-professional conflict have been said to blur the understanding of patient need in the existing multidisciplinary care team organisation (Cowley, 1999). Stokes (1984) argues that multi-professional teams frequently have difficulty working out a coherent shared purpose in practice, since members have different training which has given them different values, priorities, and preoccupations. A lack of understanding between professional groups in the multidisciplinary team about each other's roles and potential contributions to patient care inhibits the effective working of the team. Aitken and Jellicoe (1996), however, argue that the differences between health professions can be advantageous in facilitating greater self-esteem, knowledge, and respect for other professionals' viewpoint. This view is supported by Gorman (1998), who advocates working with the *strength of difference* in a multidisciplinary team. But first it is necessary to recognise where the differences lie.

Teams can be either unidisciplinary, multidisciplinary, or interdisciplinary and may or may not be integrated. The multidisciplinary team has members who bring their own expertise to the care and treatment of patients. However, these teams are not necessarily well integrated. According to Gage (1994), an interdisciplinary team is needed for patients whose condition requires an integrated approach combining the expertise of professionals from different disciplines. Integrated teams may be unidisciplinary, for example, nursing teams in primary health care comprising community nurses, health visitors, and school and practice nurses. The different skills in these teams are interdependent and this encourages the notion of co-responsibility among team members. The philosophies, relationships, communication systems, and working practices will differ among these types of teams and any of these elements can create barriers to developing practice. Likewise power sources in these teams will differ and can be a major source of tension, although the power dynamics will be more magnified in multi-disciplinary teams.

The solidity and maturity of the team, of whatever type, will determine the degree to which innovation and change are received and supported. How can we ensure that those in a team who wish to develop practice, to take a change forward, are identified? If the team does not have a strong sense of identity this can be a problem. Potential barriers within the team may also include ineffective communication, how team members relate to each other, and a lack of understanding of each other's strengths and weaknesses. Strong leadership, facilitation, mutual respect, a common philosophy, common goals, and a collective vision are all key factors, particularly as team members change and consequently the dynamics of the team also change. If new team members are not adapted to, ongoing practice development initiatives may be compromised as changes in the team dynamics engulf motivation, commitment, and potentially the leadership.

The size of the team and the care setting in which the team functions can be a barrier in developing practice, since more difficulties may arise the greater number of people who need to be involved and develop ownership, cohesion, and integration. Arguably, there is a greater challenge to how people relate and communicate among a large, diverse group in a primary health care setting that is geographically spread than in, for example a hospital ward. Practice development in the future will increasingly encompass a range of partnerships and agencies serving health communities, which can bring additional problems. The quality of the leadership, the team philosophy, and common goals are influential in bringing the team together or underpinning and supporting developments at an individual or team level.

Finally, support from the wider organisation is vital in recognising that the team is part of a whole system, since a further challenge and potential barrier for teams is the calculated risk taking encompassed in developing practice to enhance patient care. Such risk taking, set in an ethical decision-making framework with strong leadership, is crucial to developing practice at all levels. Merritt (1996) argues that each of the stakeholders involved in health care, including patients and carers, may have a different perspective on any ethical dilemma and that htis requires the acquisition and sharing of risk. She goes on to question whether we should encourage risk taking at all? The need for risk management, proceeding in an informed way, is therefore crucial. How will this done by a team or an individual within a team? Firstly, acknowledging that the individual or the team does not function in isolation but is part of a whole system will go some way to achieving change. Secondly, it should be acknowledged that the whole system exists in order to meet the needs of the patient.

## CONCLUSION

There is a diverse range of barriers to developing practice, of which we have considered only a few. One of the key challenges in anticipating and overcoming these barriers is to prioritise needs. Prioritising is about balancing all of the competing demands placed on you the practitioner or the clinical team. Prioritising is not a linear process. It is dynamic and multifaceted and runs concurrently with developing practice. Having clear and transparent goals and values geared to the patient/user makes it easier to prioritise and to keep the focus on improvements that can be made to patient care, starting from the needs of the patients. The following questions and activities are intended to help you identify and explore the barriers in your own area, in relation to systems, leadership, teamwork, and patients/users. The next chapter will help you consider ways to overcome these barriers.

◀ **Key points**

- Develop a whole systems mind-set in order to work across professional organisations and boundaries.
- Recognise organisational learning.
- Acknowledge occupational cultures and a need to see the other view.
- Organisations are messy and this mess is important to success.
- The organisation is a living whole system.
- Place value on formal and informal relationships.
- There is a need to understand culture.
- Develop a culture of empowerment.
- Aligning strategy to culture is required to achieve the strategy.
- Establish direction and motivate, inspire and align people.
- A lack of strong leadership is a barrier.
- The leader needs to be suited to work with complexity and uncertainty.
- Transformational leadership is consistent with the pre-requisites for developing practice.
- Intuition informs decision making.
- There is a need to think outside of the box.
- A range of skills are required for effective leadership.
- Make team members valuable contributors and trust them.
- Develop individuals to their full potential.
- Co-responsibility and collective intelligence of team members allows organisations to focus on the needs of patients/clients.
- Uni-disciplinary practice development can restrict or limit the impact and subsequent benefit to patient care.
- Work with the strength of difference in the multi-disciplinary team.
- Differences and power relationships between disciplinary groups can be a barrier to adapting to changes in team members.

- Practice development across agencies presents greater challenges due to different organisational cultures.
- Support from the top of the organisation is required.
- Recognise the politics and identify resources required.
- There is a need to involve and engage with patients and users in a meaningful way.
- Manage the risks inherent in developing practice.

## A GUIDE TO ADVANCING PRACTICE AND PRACTICE DEVELOPMENT

In order to help you identify some of the potential barriers to the effective development of practice a number of questions have been identified. You may find it useful to ask the questions in relation to your specific development. This guide explains why we feel these are important areas to explore before implementing your innovation or development.

### What is driving this change?

It is important to understand where the driver for this particular change is coming from. Is it being driven nationally, organisationally, or locally? Determining this will allow you to assess where the ownership of this particular initiative lies and therefore how much say you are likely to have.

### What is the scope of this development?

Understanding the size of the development is crucial and will have an impact upon the resources needed. The scope of the development should include the following:

- Is it confined to one clinical area or does it involve a number of areas?
- Is it confined to one organisation or does it cross organisational boundaries?
- What professional groups will it involve?
- How will patients/users need to be involved?

### What does the evidence say?

Understanding the evidence base for the development is very necessary. This should include evidence from previous research both inside and outside the organisation as well as data available from internal audit. If there is little evidence available then questions should be asked about how the evidence is going to be generated.

### What does intuition say about the logic?

As well as considering the scientific evidence, intuition also has a part to play. Intuition can be defined as 'understanding without rationale', Benner and Tanner (1987). Intuition is one of many tools to be used when making important decisions. Therefore, when scientific evidence or facts are lacking, McCutcheon and Pincombe (2001) highlight research evidence that acting on intuition is associated with positive behaviour and when intuition is ignored things go wrong.

## How will you know when you have achieved your goal?

Involving patients and users to give feedback on the success of the project is crucial. Questions should be asked about how patients and users will be engaged in a real way rather than the token approach that sometimes occurs.

## What are the anticipated pitfalls/obstacles?

This question needs to focus on whether the whole system and all the relevant stakeholders have been considered. Working in this way requires the direct participation of those involved. Identifying those key individuals who have an interest in your development as well as those who have the ability to influence what you are doing can be useful in identifying the people that you must communicate with.

## How will you recognise problems and how can you overcome them?

Maintaining networks of communications and connections is vital to early recognition and resolution.

## What resources are required?

Careful consideration of the resources required is vital.

### Time

How much time will be needed to undertake the development? Often teams work better when time is limited or deadlines are tight, for this creates a critical mass in terms of creativity, innovation, team cohesion, overcoming barriers, communication, and mutual support in the pursuit of a common goal. Achieving the goal within the time limit binds the team together. Will additional time be required? How many people will be involved, directly and indirectly. What time demands will be made on them?

### Logistics

How will you bring people together? Where will you get together? When? Multi-agency developments always take longer.

### Skills and expertise

Will you need to recruit or buy in additional expertise or is the expertise already available within the team or organisation?

### Funding

Do you require financial support? Is this for the development itself, to buy additional resources, or to fund staff development? What sources might you obtain funding from, inside and outside the organisation?

### Who is the manager?

An important person with respect to resources (Gorman, 1998).

### What is the skill mix of the team to take the development forward?

It is essential to know the current abilities in the team and to understand the differences among the members. What skills and knowledge does the team have? What do they need? How can the skills and knowledge be developed? Who are the leaders, the innovators, the creative thinkers? How do they perform under pressure? The following questions are derived from Gorman (1998) and West and Slater (1996). Does the team:

- Have a clear sense of team identity?
- Have clarity of roles and responsibilities?
- Have a sense of collective responsibility?
- Have clear goals?
- Know where the patient fits within the team?
- Know how people relate to each other?
- Know who is in the team and who is outside the team?

### Who are the change agents?

Understanding who the change agents are in an organisation or team is vital to initiating and sustaining practice development.

- How will you identify them?
- How will they be supported and developed?

### What is the vision?

The ability to articulate and communicate a clear vision of the development and where it fits with the wider vision is essential, regardless of the level at which the change is occurring in the organisation.

- How will the vision be developed?
- Is it a collective vision?
- Is there ownership of the vision?
- Does everyone involved understand the vision?
- How will the vision be communicated?

### Is there passion in the team to take the development forward?

Passion in the team is an essential ingredient for taking the development forward.

- Is the passion for the development confined to the leader? How will you know?
- How will the passion be developed in others?
- How can you influence others to accept your way of thinking?

- Are there others outside the team who need to become passionate about the development in order to ensure its success?

When the passion becomes contagious rather than confined to the leader or a few members of the team, mutual encouragement will help maintain the momentum.

## What partnerships are required for this development?

The scale of the change will determine the nature and extent of the partnerships you need to develop; these may be with individuals not directly involved.

- Is partnership required with individuals, other disciplines, other teams, patients and/or users, other services, and/or other agencies?
- What collaborative activity must be undertaken with these partners for the change to be successful?
- Is the partnership of mutual benefit to all partners?
- How will the differences between the partners be managed?

## What relationships need to be established to make the development successful?

It is advantageous to identify the individuals and groups that you need to build a relationship with.

- Who will you need to work with in order to plan the change, implement it, and sustain it?
- Remember that the relationships you establish at the implementation stage will not always have been predictable at the outset.
- If funding sources or specific resources are used, maintain close relationships with your contacts in these areas.

## How are you going to communicate?

Understanding the communication networks, both formal and informal, in your team and organisation is essential at the outset.

- How will you build up your communication network?
- What methods will you use? What is the most efficient and reliable? Consider multiple methods and maintain a variety.
- How will you communicate outside your organisation?
- Will you utilise existing channels of communication or develop additional ones?
- How much face-to-face contact will you need?
- How will you balance gaining information, sharing information, and giving information?
- Who are the key players you should be communicating with?

Below are a number of activities you can undertake that can help in identifying or inform you about the potential barriers in developing practice in your area. You will need to locate some of the tools associated with the activity from the primary sources suggested or undertake further searching of the literature to select something that better fits your requirements.

## Activity 5.1 – Teams and teamwork

Team Health Audit (Henley Management Centre) – is the team innovative and creative or traditional in its approach to resolving problems?
Ward Atmosphere Scale – to gain insights into staff views
Team culture – to identify ritual symbols and myths
Team parameters – who is in the team and who is the leader? (Gorman, 1998)

## Activity 5.2 – Whole systems

Whole systems event for the multi-professional team (King's Fund)
Network mapping (include patients) – who do you need to link with?

## Activity 5.3 – Involving patient and users

Process review, empowerment
Pathways of care, patient focused and friendly, evolving, patients recording variances, patient-held records

**REFERENCES**

Agor, W. H. (1986) Intuition: the new management tool. *Nursing Success Today* 1, 23–24.

Aitken, V. and Jellicoe, H. (1996) *Behavioural Science for Health Professionals*. Saunders, USA.

Bass, B. M. and Avolio, B. J. (1993) Transformational leadership and organisational culture. *Public Administration Quarterly*, Spring, 113–121.

Benner, P. and Tanner, C. (1987) Clinical judgement: how expert nurses use intuition. *American Journal of Nursing* 87, 23–31.

Cowley, S. (1999) *Nursing in a Managerial Age*. Blackwell Science, Oxford.

Deigling, P., Kennedy, J., Hill, M., Carnegie, M. and Holt, J. (1998) *Professional Subcultures and Hospital Reform*. Centre for Hospital Management and Information Systems Research, University of New South Wales, Sydney.

Dubrin, A. J. (2001) *Leadership, Research Findings, Practice and Skills*, 3rd edn. Houghton Mifflin, Boston, USA.

Edwards, M. and Hale, N. (1999) Opportunities in a managerial age. In Norman, I. and Cowley, S. (eds), *Nursing in a Managerial Age*. Blackwell Science, Oxford.

Gage, M. (1994) The patient driven inter-disciplinary care plan. *Journal of Nursing Administration* 24(4), 26–35.

Goddard, A. and Lenhardt, V. (1999) *Transformational Leadership: Shared Dreams to Succeed*. Palgrave, Basingstoke. Translation by Macmillan Publishers.

Gorman, P. (1998) *Managing Multi-disciplinary Teams in the NHS*. Open University Press, UK.

Hofstede, G. (1991) *Cultures and Organisations: Software of the Mind*. McGraw Hill, Maidenhead.

Kotter, J. P. (1990) *A Force for Change: How leadership differs from management*. Free Press, USA.

Lewin, K. (1951) Cited in McPhail, G. (1997) Management of change: an essential skill for nurses in the 1990s. *Journal of Nursing Management* 5, 199–205.

McCormack, B. (1999) Towards practice development: a vision in reality or a reality without a vision? *Journal of Nursing Management* 7, 255–264.

McCutcheon, H. H. I. and Pincombe, J. (2001) Intuition: an important tool in the practice of nursing. *Journal of Advanced Nursing* 35, 342–348.

Merritt, H. (1996) Managing risks: the ethical dimension. *Health Care Risk Report*, February, 19–21.

Miller, V. G. (1995) Characteristics of intuitive nurses. *Western Journal of Nursing Research* 17(3), 305–316.

Mintzberg, H. and Jorgensen, J. (1987) Emergent strategy for public policy. *Canadian Public Administration*, 30(2), 214–229.

Polge, J. (1995) Critical thinking: the use of intuition in making clinical nursing judgements. *Journal of New York State Nurses Association* 26(2), 4–9.

Pratt, J. A., Gordon, P. and Planping, D. (1999) *Working Whole Systems*. King's Fund.

Schein, E. (1996) *Three Cultures of Management: The Key to Organisational Learning*. Sloan Management Review, Cambridge, Massachusetts.

Stacey, R. (1996) *Strategic Management and Organisational Dynamics*, 2nd edn. Pitman, London.

Stokes, J. (1984) *The Unconscious at Work in Groups and Teams. Individual and Organisational Stress in the Human Services*. Routledge, London.

Wallach, R. (1993) Individual and Organisations: The Cultural March. *Training and Development Journal* Feb 29–36.

Wedwenburn Tate, C. (1999) *Leadership in Nursing*. Churchill Livingstone, London.

West, M. and Slater, J. (1996) *Teamworking in Primary Health Care*. Health Education Authority, London.

## MAKING CHANGE HAPPEN: OVERCOMING THE BARRIERS TO PRACTICE DEVELOPMENT

*Angela Artley and Janice Menhennet*

### INTRODUCTION

McCormack (1999) shows that since the early 1980s practice and professional development roles have assumed increasing importance and popularity in the nursing profession. More recently, strategic documents such as *The National Plan* (DoH, 2000a), *Improving Working Lives* (DoH, 2000b), *Making a Difference* (DoH, 1999), and *A Health Service for All Talents* (DoH, 2000c) have highlighted the importance of developing the workforce to deliver the modernisation agenda. Staff should have opportunities to enhance their existing skills and develop new and better ways of working. The role of the practice development nurse is central to this.

This chapter draws on a number of practical examples from a wide range of projects to demonstrate and critically discuss how one practice development team overcame the barriers to making change happen. This team was set up in 1996 and began on a small scale, working with staff in one directorate, and then developed into coordinating and facilitating practice, professional, and educational developments to meet the overall objectives of a medical division.

### PRACTICE DEVELOPMENT: WHERE DO YOU BEGIN?

The growing literature describing practice development posts demonstrates how such roles can vary immensely. They range from working as an individual specifically designated for practice development in one department, to working as a senior nurse with a trust-wide remit for practice development. In addition, they are multifaceted, often having a variety of responsibilities. Sams (1998) identified how this diversity can create difficulties for staff when preparing for the role of a practice development nurse.

This was certainly the case for the author's practice development team. Accessing the literature created confusion about exactly where to begin. Glover (1998) states that the common theme linking all practice development nurses is that each of them act as an expert, providing guidance on the development of best practice and supporting innovation in practice development. The role is not just about ensuring that top-down directives such as *Making a Difference* (Department of Health, 1999) are implemented, but also involves encouraging and supporting projects or developments that staff have instigated. The most important thread running through all aspects of the role is facilitation. This means empowering practitioners to advance care practices and ensuring that any change is introduced in such a way that it is sustained. This concept is reflected by the Department of Health (1997), which defines practice development as 'the planned systematic process of implementing change' that focuses on the 'implementation of effective person centered care'.

## MAKE CHANGE HAPPEN: PUTTING THE SYSTEMS IN PLACE

Kitson *et al.* (1996) argue that often poorly trained or supported staff are given practice development roles without appropriate supervision, support, or a strategic view of what problems to address first. Embracing that point encouraged our team to focus initially on establishing networks, both locally and nationally. This was helpful in raising our awareness of developments, identifying individuals in similar roles, and accessing professional forums that actively disseminated practice development information. This helped us plan and shape our approach.

It is also imperative that individuals in practice development roles have an awareness of how a particular trust operates as a whole. This helps them acquire a broad understanding of health care provision and establish how the skills and resources within an organisation can be used more effectively and efficiently. Without this knowledge it is much more difficult to identify and direct practice development initiatives that have a strategic viewpoint. Sams (1998) points out how many practice development roles do not have operational line management responsibility and, as such, have limited financial and human resources to draw upon. Therefore, learning how to gather resources and expertise from others is a valuable skill to develop.

Management support is key to the success of practice development posts. Glover (1998) highlights that many posts have developed in an *ad hoc* way, and as a consequence are likely to fail because neither the post holder nor the organisation is sure about what they are trying to achieve or when they want to achieve it by. The role needs to be clearly defined by the management team from the onset. Practice development is not a quick fix and should be viewed as a long-term investment in order to ensure that any changes made are sustained.

Support systems need to be put in place which promote good lines of communication between management and practice development. This approach has proven invaluable in that it has promoted progress reviews, reflection on initiatives, and opportunities to gain advice and information about potential developments to influence strategy development and the implementation of strategic objectives.

This support was instrumental in helping our team flourish in its activities. The role can be extremely varied and demanding, requiring a variety of skills and coping mechanisms, many of which are not apparent at the outset. Continuing management support has a positive impact. The personal and professional challenges associated with engaging in such work are great. It is easy to under-estimate the amount of support that is needed to meet the challenges – a view supported by McCormack *et al.* (1999).

## CHANGING THE CULTURE

Creating a setting where innovation can take place is vital to making change happen. Practice development is not just about changing a particular practice intervention. As Fay (1987) points out, it requires a focus on changing the culture and context in which care is delivered, that is, bringing about changes in behaviours, actions, language, and attitudes that are often taken for granted. Each of these can greatly influence care practices.

Transforming culture is central to practice development. The Department of Trade and Industry (1997) suggests that an effective organisation should recognise that shared culture, learning, effort, and information are the keys to high productivity and quality. The starting point to addressing the culture of a given clinical area is to establish the type of culture in the organisation or team. The preferred culture to promote change is what McSherry (1999) and McSherry and Pearce (2002) describe as a 'constructive culture'; a culture that:

- promotes learning
- learns from experiences and mistakes
- communicates to all
- collaborates between all levels of the team or organisation
- rewards, values, and develops staff.

However, this type of open culture takes time to achieve and requires a number of steps. The first step in addressing the cultural barriers that may exist in an area involves spending time working alongside staff in the clinical setting. This helps to identify the quality of the care delivered, the working practices in place, and opportunities for development. Such an approach allows rich opportunities to engage in the constructive questioning of staff and to carefully challenge existing practices, which, in turn, begins to help staff develop their reflection and problem-solving skills.

## CREATING AN ENVIRONMENT FOR CHANGE

This process, however, of changing a particular culture requires sound facilitation skills to help individuals work together as a team to understand what they want or need to change and how they can change it to achieve transformation of practice. Stokes (1984) identified how multi-professional teams frequently have difficulty working out a coherent shared purpose in practice, since members have different training which has given them different values and priorities. This point is supported by Schein (1996), who highlights that the different disciplines in an organisation can produce a number of subcultures that are not aligned to each other.

Warfield and Manley (1990) suggest that by changing the values and beliefs of those who have experience in the clinical setting it may be possible to shape the future philosophy and objectives of the ward, department or clinical area. The exercise of developing a philosophy of care should be the first step in the process of changing culture and developing a team approach to advancing practice. This simple exercise stimulates individuals to begin to question their own beliefs, attitudes, and values and to challenge existing practices. Teams rank ideas in order of importance, which leads to a group judgment and the production of a philosophy of care. The process requires considerable time to achieve but results in a shared vision of care practices and a standard to aim for in the change process. It also helps establish any conflicting views about current practice and opportunities for developments in care practices. This process is imperative in order to identify the need for change. It inspires staff to begin to realise what developments are necessary and desirable.

## OVERCOMING POTENTIAL CONFLICT AND STRESS

However, developing a philosophy of care is simply the first step in changing the culture of a given area. Experience in using this approach can, in itself, create anxieties in some staff about their individual skills and their ability to initiate change. Staff can feel overpowered by the size of the changes recommended, or that the findings of observations and group discussions are directly aimed at their individual practices, or can show signs of resistance to the proposed changes.

The suggestion of changing some practices causes some individuals conflict and stress. Schoolfield and Orduna (1994) identified that stress and conflict result when old and established ways are changed and that a grieving process is necessary before people can let go of the past. This is similar to Schon's (1991) view that people desire a 'stable state' because it gives certainty to their lives. When this stable state is questioned they become resistant to proposed changes.

The collaborative drawing up of an action plan is the next step to help encourage ownership of the proposed changes. The building up of a joint commitment towards one particular vision is a strong test for practice development staff and requires a great deal of effort. However, it is simply not enough for people to share a common vision of a better future. They will only begin to move if they know the first steps on the way and have some milestones for the future. The plan must involve, for example, the establishment of clear project protocols with realistic objectives, named individuals, time frames, and evaluation techniques.

## OVERCOMING EMOTIONAL RESISTANCE TO CHANGE AND MANAGING CONFLICT

Making change in a health care setting is a process often complicated by resistance among those the change directly involves. The practice developer must always anticipate this. As Harvey (1995) points out, 'change without resistance is no change at all, but simply an illusion of change'. Kanter (1985) describes how resistance to change refers to any employee's behaviour that discredits, delays, or prevents the implementation of a work change. Employees may resist change for several reasons and both anticipation of this resistance and an understanding of the reasons for it are crucial to the success of the practice developer's role. Curtis and White (2002) discuss how change can provoke feelings in staff ranging from pride and achievement to loss and stress. People can resist change for a variety of reasons. For example:

- the change diminishes their power or influence;
- lack of understanding of the purpose of the change;
- distrust of the intentions behind the change;
- fears about meeting the demands the change may bring;
- limited information about the change;
- lack of ownership of the change;
- differences between the managers' and staff members' assessment and perception of the situation.

Practice developers must be able to accept resistance as a natural occurrence in the change process and to apply the most appropriate strategy to help reduce or prevent its likelihood. The authors' roles involve acting as external change agents. An 'external change agent' is person from outside the ward or organisation who takes on the responsibility for introducing the change. Their objectivity helps to facilitate the introduction of a change. We begin by assessing the situation and then plan and implement the change. To help staff accept change collectively, a simple but effect method is to encourage their early involvement in the process. However, not all changes in health care settings are facilitated by practice development staff. Below we highlight a number of methods that staff can use to help overcome resistance when introducing a change in their place of work (Parish, 1996; Curtis and White, 2002).

- Explain why there is a need to change current practice.
- Educate individuals about the need for change.
- Outline the potential benefits.
- Encourage regular, open, and honest communication systems.
- Listen to individual team members' concerns and suggestions.
- Introduce the change slowly.
- Provide regular information on progress with the given change.
- Encourage staff participation.
- Provide education and training both before and during the change.

## FACILITATING TEAMWORK

Teamwork is crucial in building a 'live' action plan. The practice developer must put sound facilitation skills into operation to help ensure that individual health care professionals come together and learn through sharing practices, experiences, issues, ideas, initiatives, and especially solutions to problems. Sound facilitation skills are required by practice developers to encourage progress into what Bennis *et al.* (1976)

describes as the 'moving phase' needed for change to occur in practice. Perlman and Takacs (1990) support this by stating that facilitation is the key to success.

From the Latin *facilis* ('easy'), it is the facilitator's role to:

- make it easy for the team to work towards their goal
- maintain the cohesion of the team
- get the most from the team.

BulletPoint (2001) highlights that sound facilitation involves five steps – illustrated in Figure 6.1. The process actively encourages ownership of the change process and if done correctly leads to the formation of a harmonised group.

Practice development projects need successful team-working if they are to succeed. It is commonly assumed that team-working occurs naturally and that health care professionals take readily to teamwork. This assumption, in our opinion, is incorrect. Individuals can often work at cross-purposes or have different values and priorities. The role of the facilitator is to help them work out a coherent shared purpose.

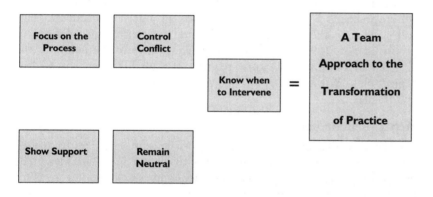

**Figure 6.1**

Facilitating teamwork (BulletPoint, 2001)

## Practice development in action. Scenario 1. Nursing Documentation Process Review Project

One of the major reasons why the Practice Development Team reviewed the nursing documentation in the Division was due to the growing variety of designs in circulation, which had been produced either in isolation or by small teams. This had led to a lack of standardisation across the Division and, in turn, created confusion for staff during the patient's journey throughout the division. This resulted in a lack of standardisation, leading to differing practices throughout the division. The United Kingdom Central Council (NMC, 1998) stresses that documentation is a fundamental part of nursing, midwifery, and health-visiting practice. It acts as a vehicle for improving communication and promoting continuity of care. However, variations in design hindered rather than helped the care process. Our role concentrated on acting as facilitators who would enable staff to acquire the necessary skills and knowledge to actively bring about change. A Project Steering Group was set up. This comprised of a number of different health care professionals of varying grades, who had been identified as key stakeholders in the change process. The group's role was to ensure rigour in the development process and that the rest of the multidisciplinary team were kept informed about progress and given opportunities to express their views.

A clinical audit exercise helped the group identify opportunities for development. The results were presented to the management team and first line managers, illustrating a multitude of documentation in use and highlighting how such variations could cause confusion for staff during the patient's journey in the division's care. In addition, the results highlighted a number of areas in which the current documentation did not meet the *Guidelines for Records and Record Keeping* (NMC, 1998).

### Step 1. Focus on the process

This initial presentation encouraged the team to tackle the problems. It is important that staff recognise for themselves what they need to address rather than having solutions imposed upon them. The discussion of the quality of documentation with colleagues was a springboard to better practice. A clear action plan was produced collectively. This addressed how the team could contribute to determining solutions to problems. Bate (1994) points out that, irrespective of the nature of the change, all development work requires the establishment of a clear project plan. Without such a framework, changes will be only tentative and fragile.

### Step 2. Remain neutral

A series of workshops were set up to provide representatives from each area in the division with an opportunity to discuss and share ideas. The group collectively examined their practices and established key areas for improvement and development. A setting was created where staff could contribute to the change process, participate in finding solutions to problems, and negotiate changes in practice. The documentation was analysed using the patient's journey through the division as the focal point.

The success of this process depended on us remaining unbiased and not allowing any one member of the team to dominate the activity. To maintain impartiality we facilitated teams in which we were not actively engaged in project work.

### Step 3. Show support

The Project Steering Group members were encouraged to develop a supportive learning environment where collaboration and teamwork were prevalent and staff were motivated to be innovative to meet the needs of the service. Constructive feedback was provided regularly and time was taken to listen to the staff's ideas and solutions. A positive attitude to the change project was created. However, Ajzen and Fishbein (1980) show that the behavioural expression of an attitude is dependent on the environmental constraints on that behaviour. A positive attitude is not the sole and sufficient motivation to undertake a change in practice if practical problems such as lack of time and knowledge are too great. Therefore, protected time was arranged to support the project and the Project Steering Group actively helped the staff get hold of the resources they required; for example, particular research material and materials to aid the documentation design process.

## Stage 4. Control conflict

The project did at times lead to conflicts in opinions and views. Professionals from different specialties sometimes had different thoughts about what they felt should be included in the assessment documentation and the design it should take. However, it is important that such conflicts are dealt with rather than ignored. Conflicts were used as an opportunity for the group to air differences of opinion and tackle problems. Such communication helped unleash ideas and innovation in the team, which, in turn, allowed the group to move on.

## Stage 5. Know when to intervene

In order to ensure maximum motivation and commitment it was crucial that the team felt comfortable that they owned the problem and its solutions. Strong facilitation skills helped achieve this. *Questioning* was used, for example, to help clarify or confirm issues: 'Is the team saying ... ?' *Suggesting* skills were adopted, for example, to help bring the team back on track: 'What about ... ?' *Directing* skills were utilised to focus the team, for example, writing on flipcharts or reiterating the key points and solutions.

Each of these steps helped direct, align, and motivate the team to design a uniformed assessment tool that was owned by the staff who would use it. Subsequently, this clear ownership of the document resulted in a smooth transition into the pilot of the document throughout the division.

## DEVELOPING LEADERSHIP

## Practice development in action. Scenario 2. Developing a systematic approach to strengthening leadership skills

This scenario describes one element of a six-month collaborative project involving the practice development team and one unit in a busy medical division. Our role during this period concentrated on acting as 'critical companions'. The project involved developing systems to help staff develop the skills and knowledge necessary for them to advance care practices in their area. The role was one of guiding, directing, and helping them build systems that would help ensure practice developments continued and were sustained once the team moved on. McCormack (1999) states that, irrespective of the source of the change, all development work should be coordinated and systematic. Otherwise change will only ever be tentative and fragile: once the catalyst for change has moved on, the development will slow down or, in the worse scenario, stop. McCormack advocates operating within a framework that recognises the complexity of bringing about change. Ward *et al.* (1998) emphasise that the process involves establishing structural and procedural support to secure advances in practice.

### Baseline assessment

The practice development team's first step involved performing a baseline assessment. This initial work highlighted several opportunities for development, one of which was the need to develop the clinical leadership of some nurses in the area. They appeared not to fully understand their role, and this issue, if not addressed, would prevent the ward manager facilitating the change process once practice development support ceased.

The change process involved implementing cultural and structural changes agreed by the multidisciplinary team, supported by research evidence, to establish new norms of clinical practice and leadership. Strategic documents such as *The National Plan* (2000a), *A First Class Service* (1998), and *A Health Service for All Talents* (2000c) highlight the importance of developing the workforce to deliver the government's modernisation agenda for the National Health Service (NHS). Clinical leadership is recognised as central to delivering improved services for patients. *The NHS Plan* (2000) highlights how strong leadership leads to innovation. Delivering this agenda requires people who can lead change with respect and dignity using both personal and position power.

Aspiring leaders need to be identified, supported, and developed. Senior colleagues have an obligation to nurture talent. They need to encourage and develop leadership qualities and skills and to create a professional and organisational climate that enables the next generation of leaders to challenge orthodoxy, to take risks, and to learn from experience. Many people confuse management and leadership; before we can proceed we need to understand the differences and relationships between leadership and management.

Andrew-Evan (1997) states that managers focus on the here and now and coordinate the 'day-to-day' operations to achieve a desired outcome whereas leaders are forward-looking and creative. Leaders have vision and direction and that direction is one in which others are influenced to follow.

Our specific aim was to develop a supportive learning environment where collaboration and teamwork were prevalent and staff were motivated to be innovative. The work involved encouraging the ward manager to adopt a transformational leadership approach to teamwork, in which management responsibilities are devolved, an open culture is generated, and decision-making and information are shared. Buss *et al.* (1994) suggest that this type of organisational culture results in improved productivity and organisational effectiveness – two important requirements if change were to progress in our absence.

We adopted what Tichen (1998a; 1998b) calls a 'critical companion' which complimented this process. In the context of practice development, the critical companion's job is to help individuals understand what they want or need to change and how they could change it to achieve transformation of practice. The role focused on facilitating the following skills:

- personal growth
- empowerment
- theoretical and practical understanding (through careful critique of practice)
- knowledge generation from practice
- transformation of practice cultures.

The project involved working with key staff one day per month for six months. Initially, the facilitation style was highly directive. It involved educational input through action learning, reflective problem solving, and role modelling.

During this period the ward manager was trained to be the internal facilitator and became critical companion to key members of the team. The aim was that this internal facilitator role would combine the role of a ward manager and project leader so as to continue the change process in the area once we had moved on. Considerable time was spent creating an open culture where decision-making and information could be openly shared and several management responsibilities of the ward manager could be comfortably devolved.

Encouraging the ward manager to work alongside the staff facilitated the process. The ward manager could help key staff develop skills of reflection in action as they delivered care, and demonstrate effective leadership through role modelling. Direction was provided to help the ward manager begin to constructively question and challenge practice to help team members develop reflection and problem-solving skills.

We promoted the use of reflective conversations; for example, 'How do you feel you dealt with that situation?' and 'What do you plan to do next and why?' This approach encouraged staff to stop and think about what was happening in their area and how their behaviour influenced practice. The process helped develop their awareness of how they currently functioned as leaders.

A series of action learning circles was initiated for key staff, which focused on, for example, challenging team members, role clarification, coordination, delegation, reflection, time management, and negotiating skills. Meetings were set up to facilitate the exchange of information, review development activities, and encourage team building.

During this period, as the ward manager's skills developed, we moved from being critical companions to working collaboratively with the ward manager/internal facilitator, helping develop skills in successful practice development.

This approach to strengthening leadership skills helped the staff understand the concept of clinical leadership. Individual and group strengths and weaknesses were much clearer, which, in turn, empowered the staff to develop their practice. The end result was a group of staff who had developed their ability to reflect on their practice and increased their confidence as clinical leaders. This resulted in an improvement in the overall leadership of the ward. The internal facilitator was now in a position to comfortably continue with the change process in our absence.

## DEVELOPING A RESEARCH-CONSCIOUS TEAM

The Department of Health document *Making a Difference* (1999) emphasises the need for practice to be evidence based. 'Nurses, midwives and health visitors need better research appraisal skills to translate research into practice ... and the capacity to undertake research.'

If we are to achieve the most for patients then health care professionals need to base their decisions on evidence. All health care professionals should be able to engage in the appraisal of evidence. However, the knowledge necessary to utilise evidence in the health care arena requires that professionals have a firm grasp of a complex knowledge base.

### Practice development in action. Scenario 3. Developing a strategic approach to encourage evidence-based practice

This scenario describes a strategic approach we put into place in one unit to help develop the evidence-based practice skills of one team of staff. During the baseline assessment stage of the project it became apparent that there was limited research activity in the unit and limited use of current best evidence to direct practice.

A series of focus groups, organised to study this issue, yielded a number of barriers to the implementation of evidence-based practice. The key barriers were:

- lack of skills and knowledge
- lack of protected time
- lack of facilities
- lack of organisational support.

A structured approach was put into place to help overcome these barriers and introduce evidence-based practice into the area. The perceived barriers listed above are not new. Such findings are supported by Hicks (1993), who found that 76% of midwives stated a lack of knowledge of research methods as the main reason for not carrying out research. Harrison *et al.* (1991) reported that nurses' tendency to implement research-based practice diminishes rapidly after qualification, since knowledge gained about the research process degrades quickly.

We firmly believe that if health care professionals at all levels are facilitated to become confident and skilled at appraising and utilising evidence, its application to practice will become embedded in their practice.

Indeed the ability to appraise evidence will then continue to develop as health care professionals progress academically and practically.

A staged approach was used and a number of workshops were developed aimed at providing staff with a framework that facilitated the development of a sound knowledge and skills base. The design addressed breaking down the barriers of research utilisation, leading to the long-term vision of an increase in practice underpinned by best evidence.

The team members who lacked the relevant skills clearly wanted to change but were not sure how to make the first step. The process involved discussions with the team, emphasising the need for their full involvement, commitment, and thus ownership of all research processes in order to obtain effective use of evidence. It was crucial for clinical staff to see themselves as key players in directing the development and evaluation of research-based evidence for practice. Organisational commitment was demonstrated by the allocation of 'protected time' for these activities and the establishment of a resource room with research material.

Bassett (1995) points out that in order to effectively utilise evidence for practice, full collaboration is required between education, management, and clinical practice teams. This is fundamental if research is to successfully underpin the development of practice. Adopting this partnership approach allowed a number of evidence-based practice initiatives to be readily put into place. Some of these are listed in Box 6.1.

**Box 6.1**

Evidence-based practice initiatives

- electronic search training
- help formulating answerable questions
- information about how evidence is generated
- critical appraisal workshops
- multidisciplinary journal club
- research methods training
- group projects
- mentorship system for project work

The mentorship system was established to enable staff to obtain guidance from an experienced researcher at any point in the research process. This helped allay fears and increase confidence to carry out a piece of research. Staff with existing research skills were used as catalysts to help generate interest in research activity and increase research competencies among other staff. This was achieved by encouraging competent staff to carry out initial projects and involving the remaining staff in aspects of the process such as literature reviewing and data collection.

Structured multidisciplinary meetings encouraged problem solving and promoted the involvement of all disciplines. Discussions among all grades of staff made it possible to explore innovations and their effect on clinical practice. This process helped motivate staff, which is important at the early stage to maintain progress.

This strategic approach helped pool people's skills and attributes and then encouraged these attitudes and skills to progress towards those required for evidence-based practice. Activity 6. 3 demonstrates one example of how we helped the team begin to develop the skills of enquiry and to explore current care practices.

## Activity 6.1

Think of an area of your practice which you carry out frequently and consider:

● Do you know for certain what constitutes good practice for that area?
● Do you have available current literature that provides evidence of what constitutes good practice for the area?
● Could you identify and obtain literature, which provides evidence of what constitutes good practice for the area?
● Could you analyse and summarise the literature?
● Could you identify from the literature what you and your colleagues could change to improve the clinical effectiveness of your practice? (NHS Executive, 1998)

The proliferation of literature available makes it increasingly difficult for staff to keep up to date. If staff enter the evidence-based practice cycle they enter a lifelong approach to staying up to date which will

**Figure 6.2**

Evidence-based practice: implementing research findings in practice

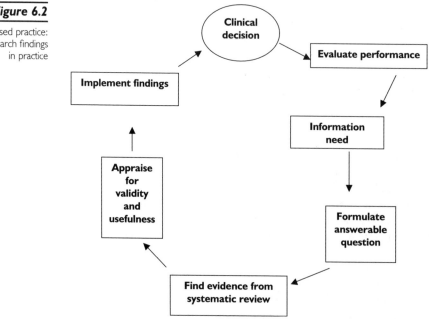

empower them with a strong combination of best evidence and professional judgment. Figure 6.2 provides one diagrammatical example of the evidence-based practice cycle that we have encouraged.

Evidence-based practice integrates individual clinical expertise with the best available clinical evidence from systematic review. It is an excellent way of staying up to date, getting your voice heard and developing professionally. However, this is not enough. Health care professionals need to work in partnership with other professionals and to cross organisational boundaries to successfully introduce evidence into practice. Teamwork needs to be strong in order to translate the evidence into improving the patient's experience.

## PROMOTING PARTNERSHIPS

Partnership is central to the government drive to modernise the NHS. This is reflected in a number of documents calling for organisations to work collaboratively for the benefit of quality services. Clinical staff are frequently what McCormack (1999) calls the 'individual innovators' who have a vision to advance practice. Often, however, these ideas go no further than the clinical area in which they were generated. Furthermore, staff who question practice are sometimes told, 'That's just the way we do things here.'

> *How do practice developers get to know about new ideas or projects?*

> *How do practice developers empower and support individuals to progress with ideas or expand projects?*

The number of practice development posts in the authors' trust has greatly increased since 1999. Developments have grown as a consequence. However, these need to be coordinated to ensure that work is not duplicated and work disseminates across the trust. Glover (1998) describes how practice development staff can become isolated in such roles. This can result in limited awareness of developments taking place in other areas of the trust.

Networks are essential to help ensure that practice development staff share innovative strategies and projects. The continuous facilitation of others to develop best practice can, at times, result in ignoring one's own development needs. Learning sets in the workplace are imperative to help support and develop the knowledge and skills of practice development staff.

Squire (2000) emphasises that learning in teams, developing multidisciplinary education and training across professional boundaries, is the way forward to creating learning environments. It will encourage health care professionals to work in partnerships in sharing ideas and solving problems that focus on what is important to the patients. How do we foster this approach of shared learning and problem solving?

### Practice development in action. Scenario 4. Working in partnership

This scenario describes one approach we used to develop successful ways of encouraging health care professionals to work in partnership, facilitate the development needs of practice development staff, capture innovative ideas, share best practice, and help turn an individual's or team's vision into a reality.

The first stage of the project involved putting systems in place that would promote practitioner-owned development work among staff in the authors' division. The project involved setting up a 'Practice and Professional Development Forum' for health care professionals with ideas, projects, or simply an interest in practice development. The specific aims of the forum are listed in Box 6.2.

**Box 6.2**

Divisional Practice and Professional Development Group

Specific aims
- Share and discuss projects
- Identify best practice and encourage its dissemination
- Look at practical ways to share and develop practice
- Encourage and support networking both locally and nationally

The project, although still in its infancy, has proved popular with diverse health care professionals. The membership is multi-professional and successes within the first quarter have included:

- A multidisciplinary poster exhibition open to all trust staff and local academic institutions. The event shared academic course work and individual and team projects.
- The production of two division-focused training programmes. The first was designed to train health care assistants to competently write objective data in nursing documentation under four specific 'activities of daily living'. The second was a Preceptorship Programme consisting of ten core competencies. These were written by various disciplines across the division.

Through the forum a safe environment has developed where staff, regardless of position or grade, feel safe, confident, and supported to explore and pursue the advancement of care practices.

The second stage of the project was concerned with creating a partnership with an academic institution to collaboratively set up an arena where staff across the trust with a practice development remit could share practices, experiences, issues, ideas, initiatives, and especially solutions to problems.

Opportunities needed to be created to bring these individuals together. Through pooling skills, knowledge, and experiences, a group can enhance the quality of care it provides. A learning set, collectively designed by an academic institution and the network members, supported the generation of knowledge and enhanced skills and confidence.

Traditionally, the relationship between practice settings and academic institutions has been that the latter produce the knowledge to be applied by the former to improve practice. McCormack (1999) describes how the creation of partnerships between such institutions creates opportunities for the generation of knowledge through practice development. This practice and professional development network group provided many benefits, some of which are listed in Box 6.3.

---

**Box 6.3**

Practice and Professional Development Network Group

*Benefits*
- Share innovative strategies and projects
- Explore issues around aspects of practice development
- Look at practical ways staff can share and develop practice activity
- Participate in action learning sets to advance skills and knowledge
- Identify best practices and encourage its dissemination
- Provide opportunities to examine approaches to practice development

---

## CONCLUSION

This chapter demonstrates the multifaceted role of practice development staff. It provides some examples of initiatives we have put into place over our first four years in post. The examples chosen were:

- changing culture
- leadership skills
- teamwork
- evidence-based practice skills
- developing partnerships.

These examples address a number of the common barriers to making change happen and illustrate the complexity of the role of practice development. However, the common theme running through all the scenarios is that success in the change process depends upon sound facilitation skills and a systematic approach. As Squire (2000) points out, learning in teams and training across different professional boundaries are the way forward to creating learning environments. They encourage health care professionals to work in partnership in sharing ideas and solving problems that focus on what is important to the patients.

Fostering these approaches makes practice development the vehicle to enable individuals and teams to achieve transformation of practice which improves the patient's experience. As individual health care professionals, we must understand the barriers and develop strategies that will not only overcome them but also help sustain initiatives. Failure to embrace the challenge will result in change that is merely tentative and fragile.

| Key points ▶ | Practice development: |
|---|---|

Practice development:

- is diverse, multifaceted, and complex in nature;
- requires cultural, organisational, and management support to create an environment in which excellence in practice can flourish;
- is based on the development of multi-professional partnerships, team-working, and requires networking, both inside and outside the organisation;
- is excellent for promoting and developing a research-aware workforce and the delivery of evidence-based practice.

**RECOMMENDED READING**

Glover, D. (1998) The art of practice development. *Nursing Times* 94(36).

McCormack, B. (1999) Towards practice development – a vision in reality or a reality without a vision? *Journal of Nursing Management* 7, 255–264.

**REFERENCES**

Ajzen, I. and Fishbein, M. (1980) *Understanding Attitudes and Predicting Social Behavior*. Englewood Cliffs, NJ, Prentice Hall.

Andrew-Evans, M. (1997) The leadership challenge in nursing. *Nursing Management* 4(5), 8–11.

Bassett, C. (1995) The sky is the limit. *Nursing Standard* 9(39), 12–15.

Bate (1994) *Turtles All the Way Down: Strategies for Change*. Butterworth Heinemann, London.

Bennis, W. E., Benne, K. D. and Chin, R. (1976) *The Planning of Change*, 3rd edn. Holt, Riehart & Winston, Orlando.

BulletPoint (2001) BulletPoint: for the Thinking Manager. Sample Issue, Why change fails: the enemies within. Bulletpoint Communications, Surrey.

Curtis, E. and White, P. (2002) Resistance to change. *Nursing Management* 8(10), 15–19.

Department of Health (1997) *The New NHS. Modern, Dependable*, CM3807, HMSO, London.

Department of Health (1998) *A First Class Service: Quality in the New NHS*. HMSO, London.

Department of Health (1999) *Making a Difference: Strengthening the Nursing, Midwifery and Health Visiting Contribution to Health and Healthcare*.

Department of Health (2000a) *The National Plan*. HMSO, London.

Department of Health (2000b) *Improving Working Lives*. HMSO, London.

Department of Health (2000c) *A Health Service for All Talents*. HMSO, London.

Department of Health (2001) *Implementing the National Plan*. HMSO, London.

Fay (1987) *Critical Social Science: Liberation and Its Limits*. Polity Press, Oxford.

Department of Trade and Industry (1992) *Partnership with People*. London.

Glover, D. (1998) The art of practice development. *Nursing Times* 94(36), 58–59.

Harrison *et al.* (1991) Changes in nursing students' knowledge about and attitudes towards research following an undergraduate research course. *Journal of Advanced Nursing* 16, 807–812.

Harvey, T. R. (1995) *Checklist for Change: A Pragmatic Approach to Creating and Controlling Change*, 2nd Edn. Technomic, Lancaster PA.

Hicks, C. (1993) A survey of midwives, attitudes to, and involvement in, research: the first stage in identifying needs for a staff development programme. *Midwifery* 9, 51–62.

Kanter, J. (1985) The purpose of change in the long term mentally ill: a naturalistic perspective. *Psychosocial Rehabilitation Journal* 9(1), 55–69.

Kitson, A., Ahmed, L. B., Harvey, G., Seers, K. and Thompson, D. R. (1996) From research to practice: one organisational model for promoting research practice. *Journal of Advanced Nursing* 23(30), 430, 440.

McCormack, B. (1999) Towards practice development – a vision in reality or a reality without a vision? *Journal of Nursing Management* 7, 255–264.

McSherry, R. (1999) Practice and Professional Development. *Health Care Risk Report* 6(1), 21–22.

McSherry, R. and Pearce, P. (2002) *Clinical Governance: A Guide to Implementation for Healthcare Professionals*. Blackwell Science, Oxford.

NHS Executive (1998) *Achieving Effective Practice: A Clinical Effectiveness and Research Information Pack for Nurses, Midwives and Health Visitors*. HMSO, London.

Parish, A. A. (1996) Managing change. *Nursing Management* 3(2), 11.

Perlman, D. and Takacs, G. J. (1990) The 10 stages of change. *Nursing management* 21(4), 33–38.

Sams, D. (1998) Reflections of a practice development nurse, *Nursing Times and Learning Curve*, January 7, Vol. 1, No. 11.

Schein, E. (1996) Three cultures of management: the key to organizational learning. *Sloan Management Review*.

Schon, D. A. (1991) *The Reflective Practitioner: How Professionals Think in Action*. Avebury, Aldershot.

Schoolfield, M. and Orduna, A. (1994) Understanding staff nurse responses to change: utilisation of a grief change framework to facilitate innovation ... introduction to patient focused care. *The Clinical Nurse Specialist*, 8(1), 57–62.

Squire, S. (2000) Clinical governance in action: part 7: effective learning. *Professional Nurse* 16(4), 1014–1015.

Stokes, J. (1984) *The Unconscious at Work in Groups and Teams. Individual and Organisational Stress in the Human Services*. Routledge, London.

Tichen, A. (1998a) Professional craft knowledge in patient-centered nursing and the facilitation of its development. D.Phil. thesis, Department of Educational Studies, University of Oxford, Oxford.

Tichen, A. (1998b) *A Conceptual Framework for Facilitating Learning in Clinical Practice*. Occasional Paper Number 2, Center for Professional Education Advancement, Lidcombe, Australia.

UKCC (1998) *Guidelines for Records and Record Keeping*. London.

Ward, M., Tichen, A., Morrell, L., McCormack, B. and Kitson, A. (1998) Using a supervisory framework to support and evaluate a multiproject practice development programme. *Journal of Clinical Nursing* 7, 29–36.

Warfield and Manley (1990) Developing a new philosophy in the NDU. *Nursing Standard* 4(41), 27–30.

# 7 THE LEGAL AND CLINICAL RISK IMPLICATIONS OF PRACTICE DEVELOPMENT

*Jean Carter*

## INTRODUCTION

This is a period of great change and opportunity for health care professionals. The Department of Health's reforms and policies (Department of Health [DoH], 1997; 1998; 2001) outline a radical programme of modernisation, looking critically at services and how they can be improved from the perspectives of the provider and user. *The NHS Plan* (DoH, 2000a) highlights many areas of development for staff, which will require changes in roles and responsibilities having significant implications for practice development. Modernisation of the National Health Service (NHS) is a great opportunity for advancing and improving practice by the creation of new roles and responsibilities and evaluating existing practices to improve the efficiency and effectiveness of the service, organisation, and outcomes for the patient/carer. In rising to the challenges of a modernising NHS, health care professions must take every opportunity to develop new and existing roles to improve patient/ carer outcomes while taking into consideration the current climate of public dismay and lack of trust following the media attention to the numerous exposures of serious incidents and poor practice.

In the midst of this we have, on the one hand, significant opportunity to develop practice and, on the other, a significant increase in patient and carer perception of what they would view as 'appropriate' care and treatment. However, to accommodate either, the health care professional must have a solid knowledge of the legal and clinical risk implications of practice development. Ignorance is no defence in the sphere of law and clinical risk.

This chapter aims to provide the reader with a minimum baseline of knowledge with sources of further reading to pursue in areas relevant to individual practice. The chapter is not intended to be a legal chapter but a consideration of the practical aspects of legal and clinical risk issues in relation to practice development. Health care professionals are encouraged to seek advice from local expertise in their own organisations about specific events and about developments in clinical practice. Although this chapter may give the impression that practice development is surrounded by risks, it must be emphasised that not to develop practice could also expose practitioners and patients to significant risk and this could progress to initiation of the legal process. The key areas considered in this chapter are accountability, clinical negligence, consent, the Human Rights Act, and clinical risk management, which are all central to the advancing of efficient and effective practices for the individual, team, and organisation.

## DRIVERS FOR ADVANCING PRACTICE: THE NEED FOR HEALTH CARE PROFESSIONALS TO HAVE LEGAL AND CLINICAL RISK AWARENESS

The drivers for modernisation of the NHS are vast, varied, and complex. Raised public expectations, increased numbers of older people requiring acute, rehabilitative, and continuing care, more complaints going on to litigation, easier access to information, advances in health care technology, and the need for evidence-based practice are to name but a few (McSherry and Pearce, 2002). The challenge and opportunities facing the government, NHS, the professions, and individual health care professionals are in responding to these drivers. The way forward is to develop new and evaluate existing practices in order to provide continuous quality improvements and efficient and effective outcomes. The latter may be achieved by the creation of new opportunities and roles for health care professionals to facilitate innovative ways of providing health care. As outlined in Chapter 2, practice development is an ideal catalyst of response to such a challenge.

## Activity 7.1 _____

On a sheet of paper note down the recent government reforms or policies that you have read or discussed with other colleagues which are related to legal or risk management issues.

For more information read on and compare your findings with those outlined in the chapter.

The government realises the potential in enhancing the roles and responsibilities of the professions to enhance the delivery of clinical services along with raising their awareness of the legal and risk management issues attached to such developments, and has published a number of significant policies (Box 7.1).

**Box 7.1**

Policies and reforms that seem to be directed towards reducing clinical risks by improving the quality of services and career pathways and opportunities for NHS Staff

*The White Papers* Modern, Dependable *(DoH, 1997) and* Quality in the New NHS *(DoH, 1998)*

Introduction of 'clinical governance' could be viewed as a response by the government to concerns about the ways health care professionals govern their clinical practice and to deal with the drivers outlined above (NHS Executive, 1999).

*The report* An Organisation with a Memory *(DoH, 2000b)*

This raises issues related to adverse health care events and near-miss adverse health care events in clinical practice, with ten recommendations for improvement. The significant change is the development of a National Incident Reporting System in order to share meaningful data and lessons learnt across the NHS.

Building a Safer NHS for Patients *(DoH, 2001b)*

This sets out the government's plans for promoting patient safety by focusing on actions needed to develop a system to learn from events across the whole of the NHS. The document introduces the new independent body, the National Patient Safety Agency, that will implement and operate the system with one core purpose – to improve patient safety by reducing the risk of harm through error. Practitioners should also be aware the document includes details of an improved system for handling investigations and inquiries across the NHS. This is to establish a consistent approach to investigations. Serious major system weaknesses or failure of a whole service will in the future be dealt with by only two options: an independent investigation commissioned by either the Department of Health or the Commission for Health improvement (CHI). Current approaches are varied and *ad hoc*. Specific risks are targeted for action

The National Plan *(DoH, 2001c)*

This outlines innovative ways for improving NHS services, for example via the 'Chief Nursing Officer's 10 Key Roles for Nurses', which will ultimately culminate in the development of new ways of providing services.

---

Accommodating the challenges of modernising new roles and responsibilities – such as therapy and nurse consultants, the use of Patient Group Directions, and nurse prescribing – will have an impact on the way health care professionals execute their roles and responsibilities in the future. Although the relevant professions must take every opportunity to develop their roles to improve patient care, it must be within a framework of practice development, which is a key component to advancing practice. However, in an ever more litigious society considerations must be given to issues such as accountability, clinical negligence, consent, the Human Rights Act, and clinical risk management.

## PRACTICE DEVELOPMENT AND ACCOUNTABILITY

## Activity 7.2 ——————————————————————

In relation to your clinical practice, reflect on how you would account for your actions during a typical day at work.

For more information read on and compare your findings with those outlined in the chapter.

All health care professionals must accept from the start of their career that they are accountable for their actions and may be called to account for the actions taken in a particular situation. The Nursing and Midwifery Council (NMC) *Code of Professional Conduct* (2002) clearly states the accountability of a registered nurse. In reality many nurses recognise the reality of this accountability only when asked to prepare a statement following an adverse health care event or a clinical negligence claim. The request to prepare a statement and give an account at a coroner's inquest or to attend an independent review is still viewed with surprise by many nurses. At this point the light dawns that account-ability is a reality. It is essential that such awareness is encouraged at the pre-registration stage of training and during further training and support given to nurses after they register. The nurse must also consider the moral and ethical dimensions of their actions even if there is no legal liability. Space does not allow further discussion of these issues, but the author recognises the impact they have on practising nurses. Figure 7.1 outlines the nurse's areas of accountability.

Registered nurses are accountable to the NMC, soon to become the Nursing and Midwifery Council. The NMC's Professional Conduct Committee hears cases of alleged professional misconduct and deter-mines whether nurses should be removed from the register. Nurses are also accountable to their employer as detailed in the contract of employment. Breach of the contract of employment by an act that is allegedly misconduct will initiate disciplinary proceedings, which can take place even if no other action such as police or NMC involvement is taking place. All nurses are accountable in criminal law for actions leading to a criminal offence such as murder, manslaughter, or theft. Breach of a criminal law is dealt with in a criminal court. Some cases involve both criminal and civil law. A breach of civil law is actioned in a civil court and may not be a crime. The most common civil action is the tort of negligence.

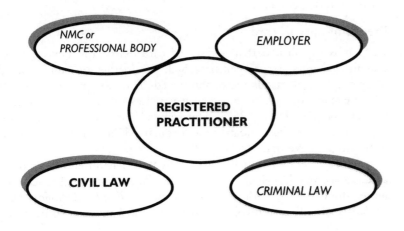

**Figure 7.1**

Accountability of a registered nurse or health care professional

## CLINICAL NEGLIGENCE

Many health care professionals are under the false impression that they will not be involved, or involved in only a superficial measure, in cases of clinical negligence. This is a false feeling of safety and all professional health care staff must be aware that they may be called to account in negligence cases. The professional will be measured against standards of an appropriate professional person. If the action in question is that of a duty normally carried out by a doctor then the standard is that of a doctor performing the action. Those professionals who would normally perform the action set the standard.

The information to establish the standard may be provided by expert evidence from a health care practitioner. Patients have the right to receive a reasonable standard of care. If this is not provided then the person can receive compensation on proof of a civil wrong, which is known as a 'tort'. A common tort that health care professionals come across is that of negligence, usually termed 'clinical negligence'. Negligence in law arises when a duty of care is broken and causes reasonably foreseeable harm.

### Duty of care

In a clinical negligence claim the claimant must prove that a duty of care was owed in the particular situation. This is fairly easy to establish in cases involving your immediate employment situation but become complex when they involve situations outside your immediate sphere of work. The legal test of whether a duty of care exists is laid down in the famous case of *Donoghue* v. *Stephenson* (1932). This case involved a person buying a bottle of ginger bear and discovering the decomposed remains of a snail in the bottle when part of the drink had been consumed. In this case Lord Atkin stated that if you can reasonably foresee that your acts or omissions could injure or affect someone close by, then a duty of care exists. In simple terms, if as a practitioner you can see that your actions or omissions are reasonably likely to cause harm to those in close proximity or directly involved then a duty of care exists to those people.

### Breach of duty of care

Once it is established that a duty of care exists, the next step is to establish whether it has been breached. To do this, one must establish what standard of care is reasonably owed. The test applied to ascertain that the standard of care expected was reasonable is the case of *Bolam* v. *Fiern Barnet HMC* (1957). The standard of care that patients can expect is that of 'the standard of an ordinary skilled man exercising and professing to have that special skill'.

In more recent cases it has been accepted that different practices in care are acceptable, which makes the task of agreeing negligence a little more difficult. The *Maynard* v. *West Midlands Regional Health Authority* (1984) case involved a patient, who happened to be a nurse, with a potential diagnosis of either TB, which was the more likely, sarcoidosis, carcinoma, or Hodgkin's disease. As Hodgkin's disease is fatal, the physician and surgeon involved decided not to wait several weeks for the results of a sputum test and performed the operation of mediastinoscopy to provide a biopsy. A risk of this type of surgery is laryngeal nerve damage, which unfortunately occurred. The patient had a negative biopsy result and was later diagnosed as having TB.

In this situation the House of Lords ruled that it was acceptable to have different opinions and practices. 'It was not sufficient to establish negligence for the claimant to show that there was a body of competent professional opinion that considered the decision was wrong if there was also a body of equally competent professional opinion that supported the decision as having been reasonable in the circumstances.' This means that if the health care professional is able to obtain expert evidence that supports their actions, then the judge faced with two conflicting responsible bodies of medical opinion should find against the claimant and in favour of the defendant. In the recent case of *Bolitho* v. *Hackney Health Authority* (1997) both the Bolam and Maynard rulings were approved. In this case the House of Lords emphasised that the use of adjectives like those used in the *Bolam* and *Maynard* cases, such as 'responsible', 'reasonable', and 'respectable', showed that the court had to be satisfied that the exponents of the body of opinion relied upon could demonstrate that such opinion had a *logical* basis.

## Reasonable foreseeability

A further criterion considered in clinical negligence claims is that of 'reasonable foreseeability'. Precautions can be taken only against reasonably known risks. Where the risks are not known a practitioner cannot be found negligent. Once the risks are known a claim arising from a second similar event has a much better chance of success. The case of *Roe* v. *Minister of Health* (1954) involved an ampoule of local anaesthetic that was stored in phenol to sterilise it before spinal injection. The ampoule contained invisible cracks that allowed seepage of phenol into the ampoule, which caused paralysis when injected into the patient. Lord Denning stated of this case that it is so easy to be wise after the event and to condemn as negligence that which was only misadventure. Lord Denning went on to say that the benefits of medical science are only achieved by taking considerable risks and that we cannot reap the benefits without taking the risks. Every advance in technique is also attended by risks and he referred to the fact that health care practitioners learn by experience and that experience often teaches in a hard way.

The one important exception to the rule that the harm resulting from the breach be reasonably foreseeable is that of 'you take your plaintiff as you find them'. A nurse might make an error that in most patients would not cause harm, e.g. intravenous injection of the wrong drug, but the patient has a severe reaction (not a known allergy) to this particular drug and suffers respiratory arrest with long-term damage. In this situation the nurse could not have predicted the serious outcome of their actions but in this case would be liable for the damage based on the 'you take the plaintiff as you find them' doctrine.

Though we would all accept that unknown risks cannot be foreseen and therefore cannot be attributed to negligence, we can challenge the failure to learn from experience. Serious examples of lack of learning are the serious, often fatal events caused by spinal injection of vinca alkaloids used as chemotherapy treatments. Since 1985, 12 of the 13 reported incidents of maladministration of intrathecal drugs involve the vinca alkaloids (vinblastine, vincristine, vindesine). Ten of these incidents are known to have been fatal; the final outcomes of the other two are unknown. In early 2002, a further case involving an adolescent was in the press.

The deaths or severe damage involve children or young adults as they are the main patient groups requiring intrathecal chemotherapy. Stringent procedures, changes in the packaging of drugs, and publication of warnings have not resolved this issue. In *An Organisation with a Memory* (DoH, 2000b) 'one of the four specific aims recommended for urgent attention' is that of reducing to zero, by 2001, the number of patients being killed or paralysed by maladministered spinal injections.

Health care professionals must accept that risks exist and that professional judgment is often required to balance the risks in any given situation. A culture that supports professionals is essential. Provision of clinical supervision and encouragement of reflective practice is important as nurses develop their roles, become autonomous in decision-making, and initiate care and treatment plans for patients.

### Causation

'Causation' refers to a causal link between the breach of duty of care by the health care practitioner and the harm suffered by the plaintiff. An example would be a drug error occurring in a terminally ill patient who dies shortly afterwards. The claimant would have to prove with factual evidence that the breach of duty (the drug error) caused the harm suffered by the patient (death). Although causation may not be proved and hence a negligence claim would not succeed, further action may be taken by the employer or relevant professional body, depending on the circumstances.

This is a good point at which to consider the 'no blame' approach when errors occur and the systems approach to accidents/incidents, which looks at systems instead of blaming individuals. This is a finely balanced issue in the health care arena and some would state that a total 'no blame' culture is not possible, but most would support a 'fair and just' culture. We will debate this issue later in the chapter but it is worth your consideration at this point.

### Vicarious liability

There are two forms of liability in relation to negligence claims facing NHS or private health care organisations. The NHS or private health care organisation that employs you has:

- direct liability where the organisation itself is at fault;
- vicarious liability where the organisation is responsible for the faults of its employees.

For health care professionals with joint contracts and/or undertaking duties in other organisations it is very important they have an explicit understanding of who is their employer, since this is crucial to vicarious liability. The nurse must also be very clear about what they are employed to do. If they take action that may cause harm and result in a negligence claim the claimant must be able to establish the nurse was an employee at the time of the incident and that the actions took place during the course of the nurse's employment for vicarious liability to be enacted. If you perform duties that are not viewed to be part of your role then vicarious liability will not apply. You may be the subject of the claim.

## Claims process

Although it is not necessary for practising nurses to be familiar with the detail of the process, it is helpful to be aware of the Woolf reforms and the associated timescales. The nurse may be required to prepare a statement and meet with the trust's legal representatives if involved in a claim. In April 1999 new Civil Procedure Rules came into force based on the report into civil justice led by Lord Woolf (1996).

In a nutshell the reforms aim to speed up the process, make the process understandable and responsive to users, establish a predictable and effective service, treat litigants fairly, and obtain a fair result. From the nurse's perspective one important change is that of the Pre-action Protocol (1998) in relation to clinical negligence claims.

Lord Woolf identified that the pre-action stage of litigation was a slow and expensive process in clinical negligence claims. As a result of Lord Woolf's 'Access to Justice' inquiry a multidisciplinary body, the Clinical Disputes Forum, was established in 1997. The Forum brings together the key stakeholders involved: Royal Colleges, Law Society, barristers, General Medical Council, NHS Litigation Authority, Victims of Medical Accidents, etc.

One of the first developments from the Clinical Disputes Forum was the Pre-Action Protocol. The Protocol aims to restore the relationship between the patient and health care provider, which is now seen by many as adversarial. It also aims to resolve as many disputes as possible without litigation. The Protocol encourages openness of communication between parties and investigation of adverse outcomes. Timeliness is a key consideration expressed by specific timescales in the pre-action process and ensuring that all parties are aware of the options available to resolve the issue. Options include further discussions or meetings between parties, mediation, NHS Complaints Procedure if explanation is sought rather than compensation for negligence, arbitration, determination by an expert, and early neutral evaluation by a medical or legal expert.

Patient suffers adverse outcome. The patient should inform the health care organisation as soon as possible.

| PATIENT AND/OR REPRESENTATIVE ACTIONS | ACTIONS OF HEALTH CARE ORGANISATION | NURSE'S INVOLVEMENT |
|---|---|---|
| Patient dissatisfied and asks for meeting and/or written explanation. | Adverse outcome reported according to local procedures. Records obtained. Investigation commenced. Explanation prepared. Meeting takes place and/or written explanation given. | May have reported adverse outcome. Could be requested to attend an interview, prepare a statement and/or attend a meeting to discuss the case. May be present at meeting with the patient. |
| Patient remains dissatisfied and discusses options with a solicitor. Solicitor requests records (response target 40 days). Solicitor instructs expert who advises on the potential breach of duty Solicitor prepares a letter of claim which is sent to the Health Care Provider. (Target 3 months for response) | Records provided. Staff informed that patient remains dissatisfied and investigations continue. Health care provider instructs solicitor and takes advice from in-house expert on breach of duty and negligence. May instruct an external expert if necessary. Case prepared ready to respond to claim | All nursing documentation will be included in the release of records. A nurse not involved in the event may be asked for expert opinion on issues relevant to nursing. If claim pursued nurse involved may be required to provide further information to legal advisor. |

**If not resolved proceedings issued and served i.e. case progresses.**

***Figure 7.2***

Practical example of the Pre-action Protocol

The Pre-action Protocol is a framework for good practice rather than a prescriptive process. Figure 7.2 outlines the process and identifies the areas of interest for nurses. This framework contains some significant points for nurses. It highlights the need for speedy reporting of adverse outcomes occurring to patients. This should be followed by investigation, interviewing of staff, and obtaining statements. Nurses should keep accurate details of adverse events that could lead to an adverse outcome. In some situations the actual adverse outcome is not seen initially but often nurses are aware of the potential and should make notes with a view that a statement may be required at a later date. As nurses' roles develop in areas such as endoscopy, nurse-led clinics, management of patient caseloads, and the roles undertaken by nurse consultants, it is easy to predict that the involvement of nurses in legal procedures will increase.

Nurses should ensure they are aware of these basic processes, including how to prepare statements that may be subject to scrutiny and cross-examination. The importance of nursing documentation cannot be over-emphasised. Documentation must be comprehensive, factual, and legible. The NMC (1998) *Standards for Records and Record Keeping* is a useful framework for nurses. Legible signatures, dated entries, details of action taken, and to whom concerns were raised are all essential. Disclosure of health care records to a patient's solicitor can be voluntary, which requires written consent of the patient or representative, or compulsory by court order. The Access to Health Records Act 1990 applies to records made after 1 November 1991. It provides patients or their legal representatives with the right of access to their health care records and the right to challenge or seek correction for inaccuracies. The Act applies to documents completed by health care professionals in connection with the care of the individual concerned. Entries before 1 November 1991 may be disclosed if the record-holder deems this necessary for understanding of the later records disclosed.

The relevant exceptions to the disclosure of health care records under the Act are:

- when the record-holder believes disclosure is likely to cause serious harm to the physical or mental health of the patient or any other person;
- when the information relates to, or has been provided by, a person other than the patient (or a health care professional) who could be identified from the records and who has not consented to the disclosure.

Nurses should consider that the documentation they complete about the care delivered to an individual may be disclosed to either the individual, a deceased patient's representative, or a legal professional. This may help focus the mind on accurate record keeping as an essential.

## Activity 7.3

Consider your own record-keeping practices. Would you alter them in any way if you thought all your records were going to be disclosed?

In your sphere of clinical practice does audit of record keeping take place?

For more information read on and compare your findings with those outlined in the chapter.

### Funding arrangements for litigation

Claimants can apply for financial assistance. The Legal Services Commission was established by the Access to Justice Act 1999 and replaced the Legal Aid Board from April 2000. The claimant applies for financial support to the Community Legal Service Fund. The Fund excludes claims for fatal accident and personal injury with the exception of personal injury caused by clinical negligence.

In some situations a conditional fee arrangement is made between solicitors and counsel. This agreement allows them to enter into a contract that provides for fees to be paid only if the case succeeds. The increasing number and expense of clinical negligence claims has called for changes in the defence of claims. Medical defence organisations have increased their premiums for professional indemnity and some offer indemnity arrangements to other professionals such as nurses. A number of nurses have considered this a requirement in view of their extended roles and responsibilities and have obtained this level of professional indemnity.

In April 1995 the Clinical Negligence Scheme for Trusts (CNST) was established as a means of pooling the costs of successful claims against NHS trusts. Membership is voluntary but most trusts are members. The Scheme pools resources, members pay a premium based on established criteria, and discount is available based on performance against the CNST Standards discussed later in the chapter. Claims before April 1995 are dealt with by the Existing Liabilities Scheme (ELS) which was established in 1996. It deals with claims in excess of £10,000.

In November 1995 the NHS Litigation Authority (NHSLA) was established as a specialist health authority responsible for initially the CNST and later the ELS. In 1999 the NHSLA's role extended to include non-clinical litigation claims against trusts, such as employer and public liability claims. The detailed management of these schemes is usually handled by Legal Services Departments in conjunction with the legal representatives of the health care organisation. It is useful for nurses to be aware of these schemes, since they may be involved in the process at some stage. Nurses will be exposed to the CNST Standards for trusts.

## CONSENT

### Activity 7.4 ————————————————————————————————

Consider your current practice and any proposed developments. Are there any issues relating to consent to medical treatment?

Are you familiar with your organisation's consent policy?

For more information read on and compare your findings with those outlined in the chapter.

This is a vast subject that cannot be debated fully in this chapter. Key issues are highlighted but reference to the recommended reading below is strongly advised. The Department of Health (2001a) has produced new guidance on obtaining consent which should be reflected in current consent policies.

A mentally competent adult has the right in law to consent to any touching of his or her person. To touch a person intentionally without consent is a tort. Battery has occurred if the person is touched; assault is where the person fears they will be touched. Obtaining consent is a fundamental part of care. Consent can be express consent, either verbally or in writing, or implied, such as attending an outpatient clinic and holding out one's arm for blood to be taken. All types of consent are equally valid but written consent is by far the best form of evidence.

Consent must be seen by health care practitioners as a process rather than a single event such as getting a form signed. The process must be based on a partnership with the patient and where appropriate their family, which includes discussion, information giving, and time to consider the information and make choices.

Consent is not a defence if a duty of care was breached or to an offence of causing bodily harm. In most clinical settings consent for operations, treatments with significant risks, and invasive procedures is obtained on standard consent forms. The DoH released examples of consent forms in 2001.

A separate consent form is available for health professionals other than doctors obtaining consent, which is particularly relevant for nurses because of changes in their role which require them to obtain consent for procedures they now carry out – such as performing endoscopies, administering complex chemotherapy, and undertaking minor surgery. Nurses must understand the principles of consent and undergo specific training if they are required to obtain consent.

## Competency (capacity) to consent

For consent to be valid the adult patient must be competent to make the decision, have been given sufficient information to make the decision, and act voluntarily, i.e. not under any coercion. Competency to make the decision means the ability to understand the information given, retain it, believe it, and use it to reach a reasoned decision. The patient might wish to refuse rather than consent to the proposed treatment. If the adult patient is competent then the refusal must be respected.

The current leading case is Re C (1994). This case involved a patient in a mental hospital with paranoid schizophrenia and who suffered delusions. The patient developed a gangrenous foot which the surgeons felt should be AHPutated. The patient refused, stating he would rather die with two feet than have the AHPutation. In this case the High Court found the patient to be competent and his refusal should be honoured. In later cases the courts have advised that when assessing competency to consent, other issues should be taken into account, such as panic, fear, pain, shock, and drugs. This brings out the complexity of consent, but nurses are often well placed to observe and comment on these factors as the patient's advocate.

## Information to patients

Sufficient information is required for the patient to give informed consent. Although informed consent has substantial foundations in law, it is essentially an ethical imperative (American College of Obstetricians & Gynaecologists, 1992). The process of informed consent involves mutual communication of information and a shared decision-making process including both the patient and the health care practitioner. The matter of how much information is sufficient is a matter of constant debate.

*Sidaway* v. *Board of Governors Bethlehem Royal Hospital* (1985) involved Mrs Sidaway undergoing an operation on her spine to relieve constant pain. Following the operation she suffered paralysis and obvious severe disability. One of the recognised risks of the operation is damage to the nerve root, which was explained, but a less common risk is that of total paralysis. Mrs Sidaway was informed of the risk of nerve damage but not that of paralysis. She stated that if she had known she would not have undergone the surgery. The court held that the surgeon had acted reasonably, since at the time of the surgery it was accepted practice not to reveal the less common risk of paralysis.

New professional guidance will influence future cases and challenge current accepted practice. More pressure is being brought to bear to explain in non-technical language the risks associated with the procedure and the other options for treatment. This is a difficult balance, since explaining even those risks that are uncommon could be seen as overburdening the patient and making the decision to consent even more difficult. Some professional bodies give explicit advice on the risks that must be disclosed to patients before obtaining consent.

There is a requirement that a health professional seeking to obtain consent must disclose what a reasonable person would be likely to consider significant in deciding whether to consent – the 'reasonable patient' test (Heneghan, 1996).

The difficulty occurs when patients do not wish to know the risks in detail. This is in a way making a choice therefore forcing information onto patients about the risks would not be appropriate. Patients are individuals and respond in an individual manner; carefully documented collaborative discussions will support the claim that sufficient information was provided before obtaining consent. Some patients find it helpful to view a model such as a catheter or artificial joint or a supporting diagram as part of the information before consent. These actions should be documented and copies of diagrams used placed in the health care records if possible.

## Emergency situations

In an emergency situation such as an unconscious adult for whom life-saving treatment is required, the doctrine of necessity applies. Treatment that is life saving can be carried out but not other procedures that cannot be deemed life saving. An adult cannot consent on behalf of another adult. If available, the relatives should be included in the discussions and this should be documented but relatives cannot give or refuse consent for another adult. The consultant in charge must apply the doctrine of necessity and not ask family members to sign consent forms. Should evidence be produced such as a valid advance directive (living will) then this should be taken into account.

If the adult patient is not unconscious but does not have the capacity to consent, then treatment can be carried out in the patient's 'best interests'. The test applied is that of *Bolam* and must be accepted by a responsible body of medical opinion.

## Children

The Family Law Reform Act 1969 gives 16–17-year-olds the same rights as adults regarding consent to medical treatment provided they are competent. The consent of a child of this age cannot be overridden by a parent. However, should the child refuse treatment, this can be overridden by the courts, parents, or those with parental responsibility if it is deemed in of the child's best interests. Children under 16 if *Gillick* competent can consent to treatment. This was established in *Gillick* v. *West Norfolk & Wisbech AHA* (1986). Though the case was about contraceptive care, it applies to consent for all medical treatments. To be *Gillick* competent the child must be able to understand what is to be done, why it is to be done, and the consequences of consent or refusal. As for a 16–17-year-old, refusal of treatment can be overridden by the courts, parents, or those with parental responsibility if it is deemed in the child's best interests. Children who are under 16 and are not deemed *Gillick* competent cannot give consent. A parent or those with parental responsibility can give consent but the underpinning principal is that the treatment is in the child's best interests. Parents who refuse treatment for the child which is deemed in the child's best interests are likely to find that the courts would rule against them. A parent cannot insist that treatment continues if it is not in the child's best interests.

## Specific issues

Specific issues such as the consent to treatment of patients cared for under the Mental Health Act 1983 and the associated Code of Practice are significant. Space does not allow for detailed discussion but sources of further reading are identified below.

Chapter 15 of the Code of Conduct gives general principles of consent and covers treatments that require consent and a second opinion under Part IV of the Act. Consent in research activities is currently being addressed via research governance processes that set out the responsibilities and standards that should be applied to innovations in a formal research context. As nurses develop their practice they may be faced with two other issues relating to consent and refusal: advance directives or statements and 'do not resuscitate' (DNR) orders.

Advance statements (living wills) can request specific treatments in the event of a loss of mental capacity. Health care professionals are not legally bound to provide that treatment if it conflicts with their professional judgment. The practitioner is advised to take the express wishes documented by a person over 18 years old into consideration when planning care and treatment. An advance directive is an advance refusal of medical treatment and is only legally binding in the following circumstances:

- the patient was competent at the time of the refusal;
- the refusal was applicable to the current circumstances (had the patient considered the situation that later arose);
- the patient had not been influenced by anyone when formulating the directive;
- the patient had been informed of the consequences of refusal.

The health care practitioner does not have to comply with a refusal of basic care such as pain relief, oral nutrition, hydration, etc. nor can they comply with a request that would break the law, such as a euthanasia request.

DNR orders are important for all nurses, other members of the multidisciplinary team, and members of the resuscitation team. Joint guidance is available from the Resuscitation Council, British Medical Association, and Royal College of Nursing (2000). Health care organisations must have resuscitation policies in place that address the issue of DNR orders and it is recommended that they are based on the combined guidance previously detailed in the text.

DNR orders have caused much media attention and concerns have been raised by patients and relatives. In summary, the orders must not be ageist or conflict with Article 2, 'The Right to Life', of the Human Rights Act 1998. The decisions made must take into account the circumstances of the individual and their known wishes.

Patients and, with their consent, relatives must be involved in the discussions, which should have a multi-professional approach and a clearly documented outcome. The use of a DNR form, which is easily recognised in the notes, is advisable with guidance on when to review the decision.

Nurses must be aware of the guidance and local procedures. In many circumstances they will be included in the discussions and will act as the patient's advocate where necessary. Challenges to both advance directives and DNR orders may be seen in the courts in the coming years and precedence will alter. Nurses must be aware of the current position and significant changes as they occur.

## HUMAN RIGHTS ACT

The Human Rights Act 1998 (HRA) came into force on 2 October 2000. It introduces much of the European Convention on Human Rights into the law of England and Wales. Its impact on the law relating to NHS care is unknown but it will bring challenges to aspects of NHS care delivery and practice.

The HRA comprises of a number of Articles, many of which have potential impact for health care professionals. The Articles are considered later in this text. A review of current practices, protocols, guidelines, personnel policies, patient information, and service delivery arrangements should be undertaken to consider the implication of the HRA and relevant amendments should be made.

European case law indicates that to have considered the European Convention on Human Rights in relation to an issue may provide some protection against a claim. In practical terms this could be demonstrated by revising a protocol such as those used for consent to treatment and include in the revised policy a prompt to consider the HRA. The practitioner should then be encouraged to document their thought processes in relation to the issue.

Since 2 October 2000 public bodies such as the NHS are bound to act in accordance with the Convention. Individuals can go to a domestic court and argue that their Convention rights have been breached. They may also seek a remedy for that breach which may include payment for damages. It is particularly difficult to predict exactly what will happen in response to the HRA because the Convention is described as a 'living instrument'. What is considered to be acceptable today and not a breach may not be acceptable in the future. This offers little direct help to health care professionals but is something we must contend with in current practice.

Table 7.1 summarises the HRA and suggests possible areas of practice it may impact upon and actions that could be considered to integrate the HRA into clinical practice. This framework can be applied to specific areas of practice – which may be a useful exercise for practitioners.

## CLINICAL RISK MANAGEMENT

The consultation document *A First Class Service* (DoH, 1998) placed clinical risk reduction activities and critical incident reporting as vital components of the overall clinical governance plan for the NHS. Clinical risk and quality of care are closely related topics. By reducing risk, nurses can make significant improvements in the care delivered to patients. The principles are applicable to all health care settings but it is acknowledged the detail will vary. Risk management is well accepted in industrial and financial arenas, but in the NHS efforts had previously concentrated on non-clinical aspects of risk.

The main aims of risk management are to identify risks that can cause harm, to reduce the risks where possible, and to monitor the impact of the reduction plan. This is achieved by means of review cycles to update the risks identified in response to changes and development of clinical practice. In some situations it may be possible to transfer the risk by obtaining appropriate insurance arrangements. Most health care

**Table 7.1**   Implications of the Human Rights Act on areas of health care practice

| Articles | Areas of practice | Actions |
|---|---|---|
| Article 1. The Convention<br>Article 2. Right to Life.<br>Protected by law. Absolute right; only exceptions are court sentences and use of absolutely necessary force. | —<br>All areas of practice. Examples include, in obstetrics, clinical staff refusing a client a caesarean section and the baby ultimately dies. Intubation of neonates, elderly patients with complex disease, DNR guidelines. Withdrawal of treatment for patients in persistent vegetative states.<br>Breach of the HRA includes a person's acts and omissions, e.g. failure to provide senior health care professional cover for emergencies; failure to enforce compulsory treatment in mental health followed by a suicide | —<br>Review of relevant clinical guidelines, policies, and procedures such as DNR orders, Consider senior staff emergency cover rotas and arrangements for access to acute emergency care for patients at non-acute or community health care premises, e.g. minor injury clinics at a community hospital. Encourage all staff to document clearly the processes and considerations, since they will be subject to close scrutiny. |
| Article 3. Prohibition of Torture | This Article is aimed at areas such as interrogation of prisoners but it could be considered in relation to consent to painful treatment that was not fully explained.<br><br>It should be considered in mental health care regarding application of experimental treatment, and detention and treatment of patients against their will in accordance with the Mental Health Act 1983. Particular consideration must be made about the treatment of children. | Attention to consent procedures, especially for new treatments. Provide information to patients on the risks of the new treatment and be specific if not all risks are known. Provide information and time for the patient to consider the information and make an informed decision. Routine documentation of consent discussions. An audit of consent protocols may be useful.<br>A review of control and restraint procedures is suggested.<br>Procedures for treating children should also be reviewed when considering the HRA. |
| Article 4. Prohibition of Slavery and Forced Labour<br>The latter excludes military service and penal sentence, etc. | Could be applied to activities undertaken in some long-term health care facilities | Activities and tasks allocated must be appropriate, and supporting guidance for staff would assist in giving clarity to avoid breaching this right. |
| Article 5. Right to Liberty and Security<br>This article has six exclusions, including lawful detention, such as of those of unsound mind.<br>Includes the right to damages for unlawful arrest/detention. | Important in areas where mental health patients are detained against their will or where restrictions are placed on them in the community.<br>Elderly care. Any areas where forms of restraint are used. | Review procedures in mental health and learning disabilities. Review procedures where locked doors or baffle locks are used. Review guidance on the use of all forms of restraint. |
| Article 8. Right to Respect for Private and Family Life<br>Exceptions include protection of health by a public authority, interference by a public authority if it is in accordance with the law and it is necessary in a democratic society in the interest of matters such as the economic well-being of the country and the protection of health. | Most agree that 'private life' includes a person's physical and psychological integrity. This could affect clinical practice in areas where invasive procedures or births take place, e.g. delivery wards, outpatients, infertility units, GP clinics, endoscopy, surgical day units. Patients could contend that the care delivered by the health care professional lacked respect for the patient's physical and psychological status and that a breach has occurred.<br><br>Delay in providing a clinical service which has a serious impact on a patient's health.<br><br>Clinical information disclosure.<br>Often applies in employment situations. | Consider current procedure guidelines against this Article. Particular areas for attention include withdrawal of consent during a procedure such as an endoscopy.<br>Pre-procedure assessment of the patient's physical and psychological status with documented evidence of consideration of any changes during and after the clinical intervention.<br>Commissioners of health care must consider national and local provision of services for the local population. Providers must respond to Health Improvement Plans and provision of services in discussion with providers. Robust policies to protect patient information and maintain privacy.<br>Ensure robust personnel policies are in place. |
| Article 9. Freedom of Thought, Conscience and Religion<br>Article 10. Freedom of Expression<br>There are certain exceptions, such as protection of health and reputation | This is more than verbal expression: mode of dress is an expression.<br>Preparation of patients for theatre or other procedures. | Mechanisms to address these issues and make suitable arrangements before the event where possible. |

| | | |
|---|---|---|
| Article 11. Freedom of Assembly and Association<br>This includes the right to join trade unions. Protection of health is one of the exclusions. | Mostly apply to the activities of employees. | Personnel policies and seek advice if needed. |
| Article 12. Right to Marry | Mental health and learning disabilities. | Guidance available to assist staff. Access to expert advice if needed. |
| Article 14. Prohibition of Discrimination<br>This covers sex, religion, race, colour, origin, language, birth, politics, property, etc.<br>Article 16. Restrictions on Political Activity of Aliens | Any areas where decisions must be made when resources are limited about which patients should receive a particular treatment. | Robust and transparent decision-making that does not breach this article. |
| Article 17. Prohibition of Abuse of Rights<br>Article 18. Limitation on Use of Restrictions on Rights | This is used in conjunction with other articles. | |

organisations have an incident-reporting system which involves the completion of forms whose details are then recorded on a database. Regular reports should be available to your clinical area to inform the staff about the incidents occurring.

Clinical staff can easily undertake a clinical risk assessment in their area of practice. Staff simply identify the clinical risks and give them a rating using a simple risk-rating method of consequence frequency. The highest risks require action plans to reduce the risk. The action plans may include adequate monitoring equipment, staff available with the necessary clinical skills and knowledge, access to senior colleagues, or agreement of clinical guidelines. As practice develops, the need for assessment of risks is essential. This will help to prevent risks to patients and staff and reduce the number of clinical negligence claims.

A local forum should exist to review incident reports, the outcome, and lessons learnt where serious events have been investigated and feedback from risk assessments has been agreed. When adverse events do occur and require investigation it soon becomes obvious there are broader issues than those concerning the individual and the single event. Reason (1995) describes the trajectory of events as follows.

## Corporate/organisational level

A full review of the systems involved often reveals decisions made at a corporate level which sit as latent failures until further circumstances occur and an adverse event occurs. This could be a corporate decision to freeze vacancies, not to renew a service contract deemed unnecessary, or to change procedures or processes.

## Workplace

In the workplace there may be human error, such as lapse of memory. There may also be violation-producing activities, such as new targets for numbers of patients seen which do not allow enough time for procedures to be carried out properly. Excess overtime shifts can generate error-producing conditions because of fatigue.

## Individual

Errors can occur such as picking up the wrong syringe, as can violations such as choosing not to check the medication against the drug chart orthe patients identity band. In some situations corporate and workplace issues influence individual actions at particular points in the process.

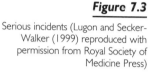

**Figure 7.3**

Serious incidents (Lugon and Secker-Walker (1999) reproduced with permission from Royal Society of Medicine Press)

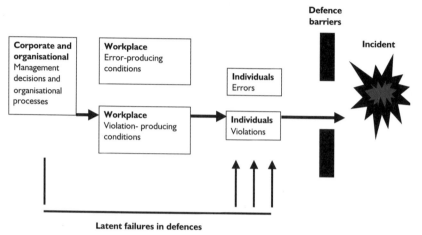

## Incident

These preceding events then breach the defensive policies and procedures that the organisation has put in place and an adverse event occurs. This is demonstrated in Figure 7.3. On an average day in health care these latent and active failures are taking place all the time but policies and procedures or personal observations intervene and the failure is stopped. But when a number of these failures line up together the normal defence barriers are breached and an incident occurs. This may be likened to multiple slices of Swiss cheese as shown in Figure 7.4.

Most organisations utilise the model of root cause analysis (RCA) to conduct reviews of adverse events. This is a problem-solving model that encourages identifying the root cause of the event rather than just addressing the initial, often superficial cause.

During 2001/2002 the National Patient Safety Agency (NPSA) arranged for a number of NHS sites to pilot an incident-reporting system that included the use of RCA models to identify the true causes of incidents. The pilot has been evaluated and national guidelines will be released by the NPSA on national incident reporting and investigation in the autumn of 2002.

To implement successful risk management programmes the staff must be clear about the repercussions of reporting incidents. Where possible, a 'no blame' culture should be in place to encourage incident reporting.

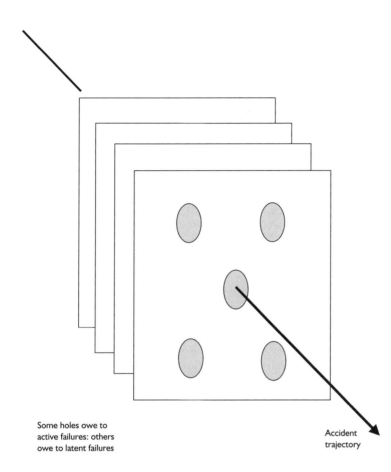

**Figure 7.4**

Breached defences: Swiss cheese model (Lugon and Secker-Walker (1999) reproduced with permission from Royal Society of Medicine Press)

Some holes owe to active failures: others owe to latent failures

Accident trajectory

A total no blame culture is deemed by many as not appropriate where there must be professional accountability. Most health care organisations have a policy statement that clarifies when disciplinary procedures may be implemented. These are usually restricted to gross misconduct, repeated events despite training and mentorship, flagrant abuse of policies and procedures, and serious criminal offences. Clinical risk data should be used to inform clinical audit activities and encourage a multi-disciplinary approach to audit. Information from clinical claims and complaints should also be considered part of the risk management activities in clinical areas, since they provide important information to help reduce and manage risk.

A number of trusts in England are now part of the Clinical Negligence Scheme for Trusts (CNST). The scheme was established in 1995 to protect trusts against the effects of the larger, relatively infrequent clinical negligence claims. CNST have established a comprehensive set of standards, which were revised in June 2000. The standards have three levels: achievement of these levels of standards brings the trust a discount on contributions to the scheme.

The standards address the areas shown in Table 7.2

**Table 7.2**

CNST standards

| | |
|---|---|
| Standard 1 | Clinical Risk Management – Strategy and Organisation |
| Standard 2 | Clinical Incident Reporting |
| Standard 3 | Response to Major Clinical Incidents |
| Standard 4 | Managing Complaints |
| Standard 5 | Advice and Consent |
| Standard 6 | Health Records |
| Standard 7 | Induction, Training and Competence |
| Standard 8 | Implementation of Clinical Risk Management |
| Standard 9 | Clinical Care |
| Standard 10 | Maternity Care (if applicable) |
| Standard 11 | The Management of Care in Trusts Providing Mental Health Services (if applicable) |
| Standard 12 | Ambulance Service (if applicable) |

Local assessment against the standards is a useful way for practitioners to consider their working practices against established standards. Application of the criteria in the standards offers the practitioner a robust structure to consider developments in clinical practice. Many of the standards can be applied generically to clinical care.

## CONCLUSION

We would encourage staff in clinical practice to maintain a consistent aim of improving care to patients through the development of practice. Issues not addressed in this chapter – such as personal professional accountability, appropriate professional regulation, and lifelong learning – bear significantly on the legal and clinical risk issues we have considered. Though they seem ominous, legal and risk activities should assist in developing an environment in which clinical care can flourish.

Having read the chapter, you may feel that risk and legal issues are detached from practice. However, we would strongly encourage practitioners to view these matters as an integral part of practice. In the early stages of practice development, at an individual, team, and organisational level, the headings discussed should be applied to the area of practice in question and the responses obtained should be integrated into the overall strategy for practice development.

**Key points ▶**

- Knowledge of legal and risk principles will assist practitioners in developing practice.
- The four areas of accountability are a reality and must be considered by all health care professionals, including nurses, whatever their role or location.
- Involvement of health care professionals in clinical negligence claims is likely to increase as their roles change and professional autonomy is developed.
- Health care professionals must understand the components of a clinical negligence claim in order to develop appropriate local policy and procedures.

- The Woolf reforms, in particular the Pre-action Protocol, have implications for nurses.
- Record keeping must be accurate, dated, signed, and appropriate. Health care professionals should be mindful that their records might be subject to scrutiny.
- Health care professionals must be familiar with the principles of consent to treatment. If they need to obtain consent for procedures they perform, they should receive specific training.
- Advance directives or statements made by patients must be considered if valid and lawful.
- The Human Rights Act is described as a 'living instrument'. Health care professionals must consider current and future policies, procedures, and treatment guidelines in relation to this Act.
- Risk management principles, including analysis of incidents, claims, and complaints, should be applied to all areas of clinical practice to assist in improving the quality of care for patients.
- Development of a whole systems approach to incident investigation will assist in moving away from a culture of blaming individuals.

## RECOMMENDED READING

British Medical Association (2000) *The Impact of the Human Rights Act 1998 on Medical Decision-Making*. London.

British Medical Association (2001) *Withholding or Withdrawing Life-Prolonging Medical Treatment*, 2nd edn. BMJ Books, London. www.bmjpg.com/withwith/ww.htm

Charles, V. (ed.) (1995) *Clinical Risk Management*. BMJ Publishing, London.

Dimond, B. (1995) *Legal Aspects of Nursing*, 2nd edn. Prentice Hall, Essex.

Dimond, B. (1999) *Patients' Rights, Responsibilities and the Nurse*, 2nd edn. Quay Books, Wiltshire.

Dimond, B. and Barker, H. F. (1996) *Mental Health Law for Nurses*. Blackwell Science, Oxford.

Foster, C. and Peacock, N. (2000) *Clinical Confidentiality*. Monitor Press, Suffolk.

Hendrick, J. (2000) *Law and Ethics in Nursing and Health Care*. Nelson Thornes, Cheltenham.

Lugon, M. and Secker-Walker, J. (eds) (1999) *Clinical Governance: Making It Happen*. Royal Society of Medicine Press, London.

NHS Executive (2000) *Resuscitation Policy*. Department of Health, London.

Reason, J. (1990) *Human Error*. Cambridge University Press, Cambridge.

Wilson, J. and Tingle, J. (eds) (1999) *Clinical Risk Modification: A Route to Clinical Governance?* Butterworth Heinemann, Oxford.

## REFERENCES

American College of Obstetricians & Gynaecologists (1992) Ethical dimensions of informed consent. *International Journal of Gynaecology and Obstetrics* 39(4), 346–355.

British Medical Association, Resuscitation Council (UK), and Royal College of Nursing (2000) *Decisions Relating to Cardiopulmonary Resuscitation*.

The Clinical Disputes Forum (1998) Protocol for the resolution of clinical disputes. *Clinical Risk* 4(5), 139–153.

Department of Health (1997) *The New NHS, Modern, Dependable*, The Stationery Office, London.

Department of Health (1998) *A First Class Service: Quality in the New NHS.* HMSO, London.

Department of Health (1999) *Making a Difference.* HMSO, London.

Department of Health (2000a) *The NHS Plan. A Plan for Investment. A Plan for Reform.* HMSO, London.

Department of Health (2000b) *An Organisation with A Memory: Report of an Expert Group on Learning from Adverse Events in the NHS.* HMSO, London.

Department of Health (2001a) *Reference Guide to Consent for Examination or Treatment.* HMSO, London.

Department of Health (2001b) *Building a Safer NHS for Patients. Implementing an Organisation with a Memory.* HMSO, London.

Department of Health (2001c) Secretary of State for Health. *The NHS Plan. Plan for Investment, a Plan for Reform.* HMSO, London.

Heneghan, C. P. H. (1996) Informed consent: recent developments. *Health Care Risk Report*, April, 12–13.

McSherry, R. and Pearce, P. (2002) *Clinical Governance: A Guide to Implementation for Healthcare Professionals.* Blackwell Science, Oxford.

NHS Executive (1999a) *Clinical Governance: Quality in the New NHS.* NHS Executive, London.

NHS Executive (1999b) *Summary Accounts 1998/99.* National Audit Office, London.

NMC (2002) *Code of Professional Conduct.* NMC, London,

NMC (1998) *Standards for Records and Record Keeping.* NMC, London.

Reason, J. T. (1995) *Understanding Adverse Events: Human Factors.* In Vincent, C. A. (ed.), *Clinical Risk Management.* BMJ Publications, London.

Resuscitation Council United Kingdom (2000) *Resuscitation Guidelines.* London.

Woolf, I. (1996) *Access to Justice*, Final Report by the Right Honourable Lord Woolf, July 1996.

---

**USEFUL WEBSITES**

National Institute for Clinical Excellence:
www.nice.org.uk.
Department of Health:
www.doh.gov.uk

# THE FUTURE OF PRACTICE DEVELOPMENT: AN AID TO MODERNISATION AND QUALITY IMPROVEMENTS

**8**

*Rob McSherry and Chris Bassett*

It is clear from the evidence forwarded in this text that the drivers for modernisation of the National Health Service (NHS) are vast and complex. Two of these are rising public expectations and lack of confidence in the NHS arising from media coverage of several major incidents and failings of systems and processes (McSherry and Pearce, 2002). To accommodate the challenges of modern 21st-century society the NHS needs to change. In this context, change means becoming more multi-professional, collaborative, community and user centred, and proactive in the way health and social care professionals, teams, and organisations are encouraged and supported to advance or evaluate practice. To become wider reaching and more community and user centred the management structures of the NHS need to focus their attention on nurturing a culture where staff are actively empowered, encouraged, and supported to become team-working focused. True multi-professional team-working will become a reality only when systems and processes are in place that support and value health and social care professionals and other staff and help them to modernise. Health and social care staff have a professional responsibility to enhance and evaluate individual, team, and organisational practices. Nevertheless, the government's health and social care reforms over the past six years have focused on improving quality by the delivery of evidence-based practice. The modernisation of the NHS is about improving the efficiency and effectiveness of services so that individual patient outcomes or the performance of individuals, teams, and organisations can be demonstrated. Health and social care professionals and services have not been left unsupported in the pursuit of this aim; a variety of new organisations and infrastructure have been introduced to support this initiative: the National Institute for Clinical Excellence (NICE), Commission for Health Improvement (CHI), National Service Frameworks, and the incorporation of clinical governance frameworks, to name but a few.

In essence 'the national institute will tell clinicians what to do, and the commission will make sure they are doing it' (Abbasi, 1999, 1476), although, according to Michael Rawlins, Chairman of NICE (cited in Abbasi, 1999), they will not be acting as a police force.

Health and social care professionals would accept the principle of a central system of setting, monitoring, and evaluating the standards and quality of health care delivered to patients in the hope of preventing the recurrence of anything like the Bristol case (*Lancet*, 1998). The difficulty facing health and social care organisations will be to ensure implementation and maintenance of the new guidelines set by NICE, and to have an efficient and effective system of clinical governance to support the modernisation described in *The NHS Plan* (Department of Health, 2000).

Practice issues to be clarified are whether:

- CHI evaluates the new guidelines at the level of the organisation or the individual health and social care professional;
- for auditing purposes the guidelines set standards for all professional disciplines regarding specific medical conditions;
- the proposed new guidelines or any other national targets established by NICE will accommodate variances associated with multidisciplinary team-working.

These issues emerge when reviewing a patient case study. For example, sufficient evidence is available to show that a patient's successful recovery from a cerebral vascular accident (stroke) requires a multidisciplinary and collaborative approach involving medics, nursing, occupational therapy, physiotherapy, speech and language therapy, dietetics, etc. There are many unanswered questions about how these proposed new structures outlined in the government's modernisation plans contained in the white papers such as clinical governance will operate at a clinical and practical level. What resources are available to support them at national, local, and individual practitioner levels? How will CHI facilitate auditing of compliance and monitor the overall effectiveness for patient outcomes?

We believe that the introduction of and investment in practice development in health and social care could enhance the quality of these structures at a local level. Practice development seems to go unmentioned in much of the recent literature or else is associated with continued professional development (CPD) and lifelong learning (LLL).

Practice development is much more than CPD or LLL. It is about creating an organisational and management culture based on a philosophy of promoting multi-professional collaboration and communication and of learning from colleagues' and users' experiences of services. This aim requires leaders who empower and encourage staff to work in teams in which they value and support each other's contributions. Quality improvements and innovation don't come cheap. They require investment in both staff and resources. How can we expect staff to practice using an evidence base if they are not research aware or do not have access to essential data? Likewise, how can we expect staff to modernise and develop *new* or evaluate existing practice if they are not supported to do so. It is easy to see why practice development promotes the modernisation of the NHS and the unique organisational, management, and leadership cultures of the various health and social care settings.

Practice development provides an ideal way to support innovation and changes in practice. This is because so often the role and responsibilities of an individual or team with a remit for practice development are linked to a unique set of principles embedded in a unique philosophy, culture, and environment that cannot be replicated elsewhere. The unique quality of the NHS and its associated organisations, services, and staff to create cultures and environments that enhance or stifle innovation could explain why practice development is difficult to describe. What is valuable about practice development and individuals or teams charged with its facilitation is the way it encourages staff to work and develop together within organisations. This approach is based on promoting team-working, multi-professional partnerships, and the sharing of practices within and between the departments, systems, and processes unique to the organisation.

'Quality improvements' and 'performance management' have now been placed at the top of the NHS agenda. Clinical effectiveness as well as cost effectiveness is to be measured against national indicators of success. We believe practice development aids individuals, teams, and organisations to accomplish these goals. This is because practice development encompasses and transcends all of the components of clinical governance: risk management, continuous quality improvements, professional development, research and development, and demonstrating the outcomes of performance. The modernisation of the NHS depends on individuals, teams, and organisations seeing the potential of practice development to promote individual and organisational quality. Evidence-based health and social care is important in supporting any innovative practice or when discussing the standard and quality of professional education or practice. Practice development empowers professionals to view and review their standard and quality of patient care along with the clinical and practice environment in which they work. In this way, practice development facilitates clinical governance at individual, team, and organisational levels.

Good luck for the future.

**REFERENCES**

Abbasi (1999) The man from NICE. *British Medical Journal* 317, 1476.
Department of Health (2000) *The NHS Plan: A Plan for Investment, A Plan for Reform*. London.
*Lancet* (1998) Editorial: First Lessons from the 'Bristol Case', *Lancet*, 351, 117, 1669.
McSherry, R. and Pearce, P. (2002) *Clinical Governance: A Guide to Implementation for Healthcare Professionals*. Blackwell Science, Oxford.

# INDEX

Page references in italic indicate figures, tables or boxes.